THIS BOOK BLONGS TO

____

____

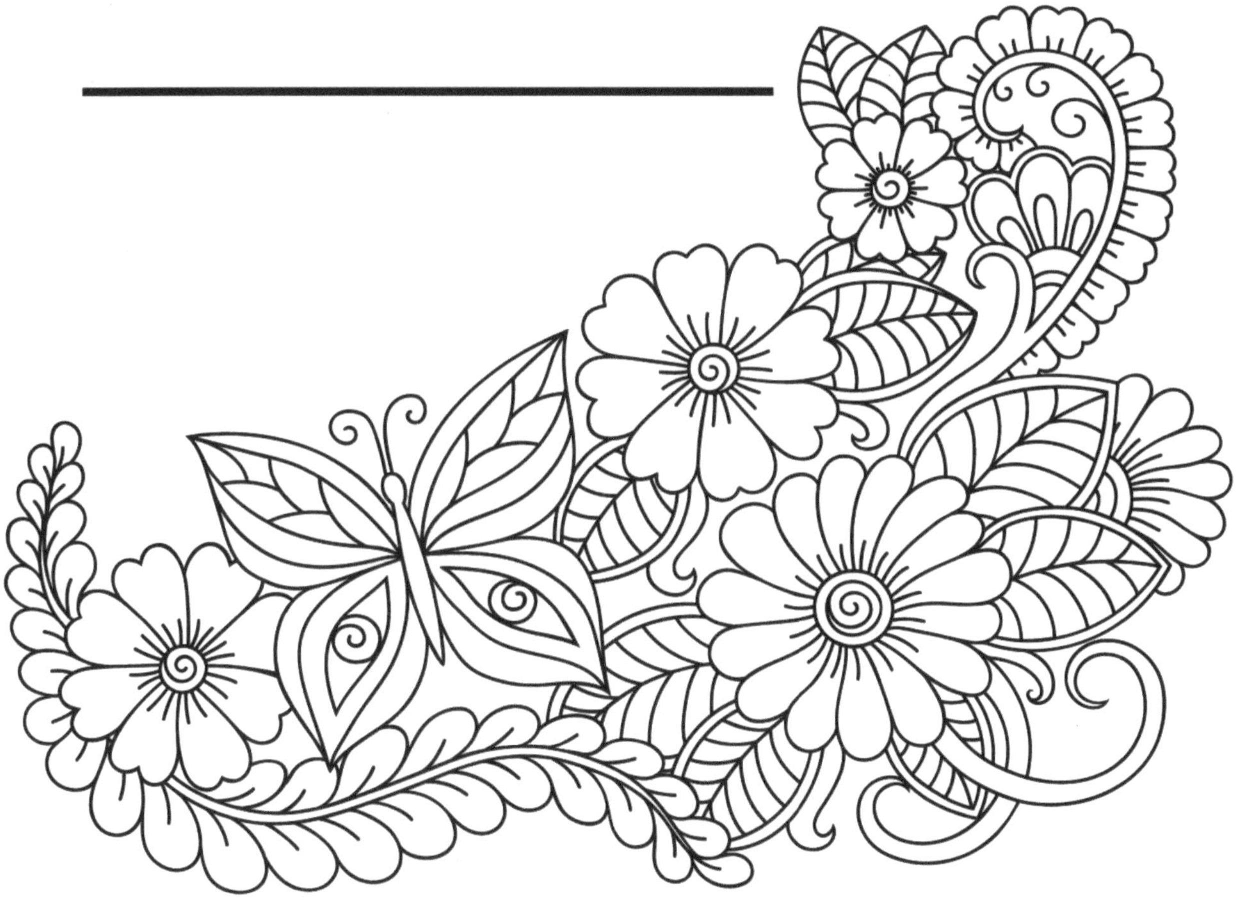

Dear stress

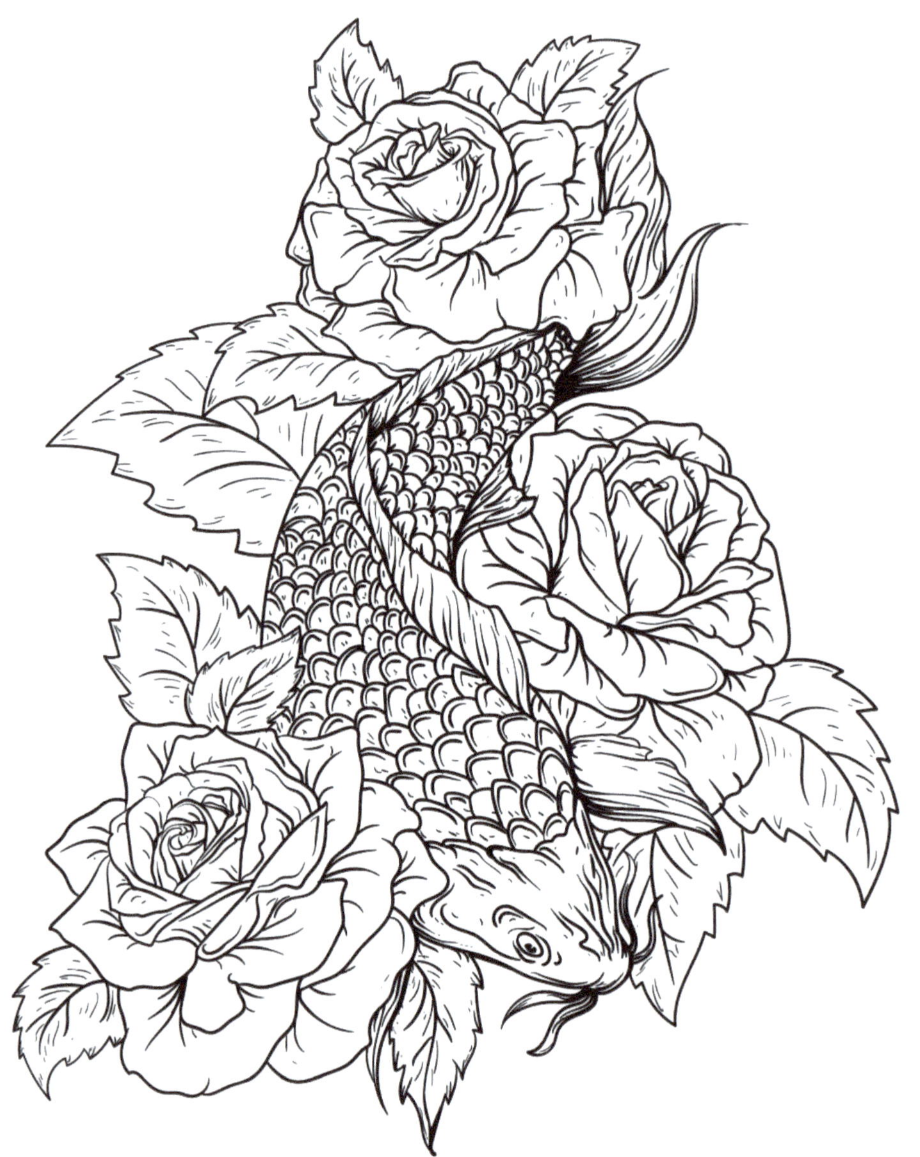

lets breakup

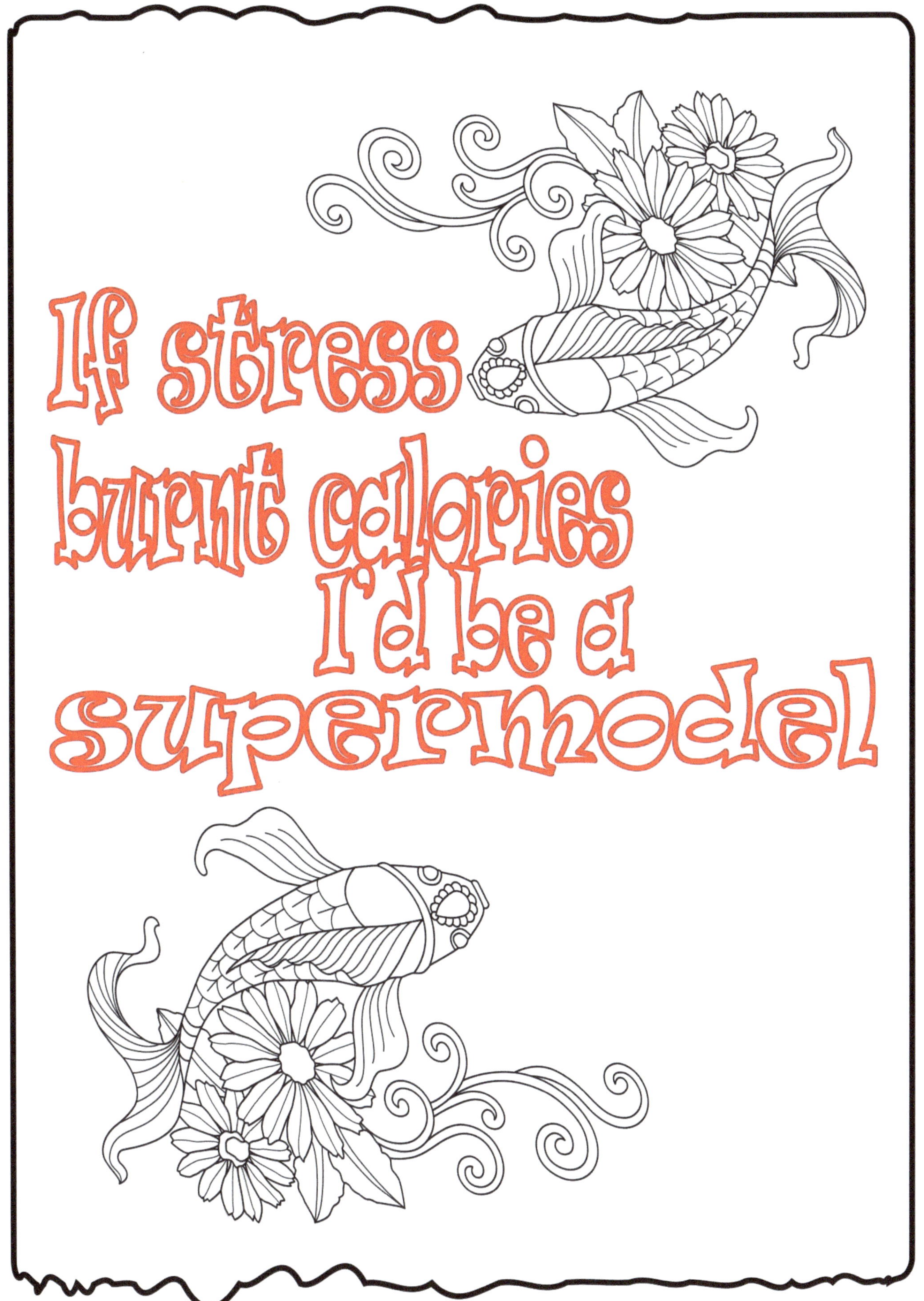

If stress
burnt calories
I'd be a
supermodel

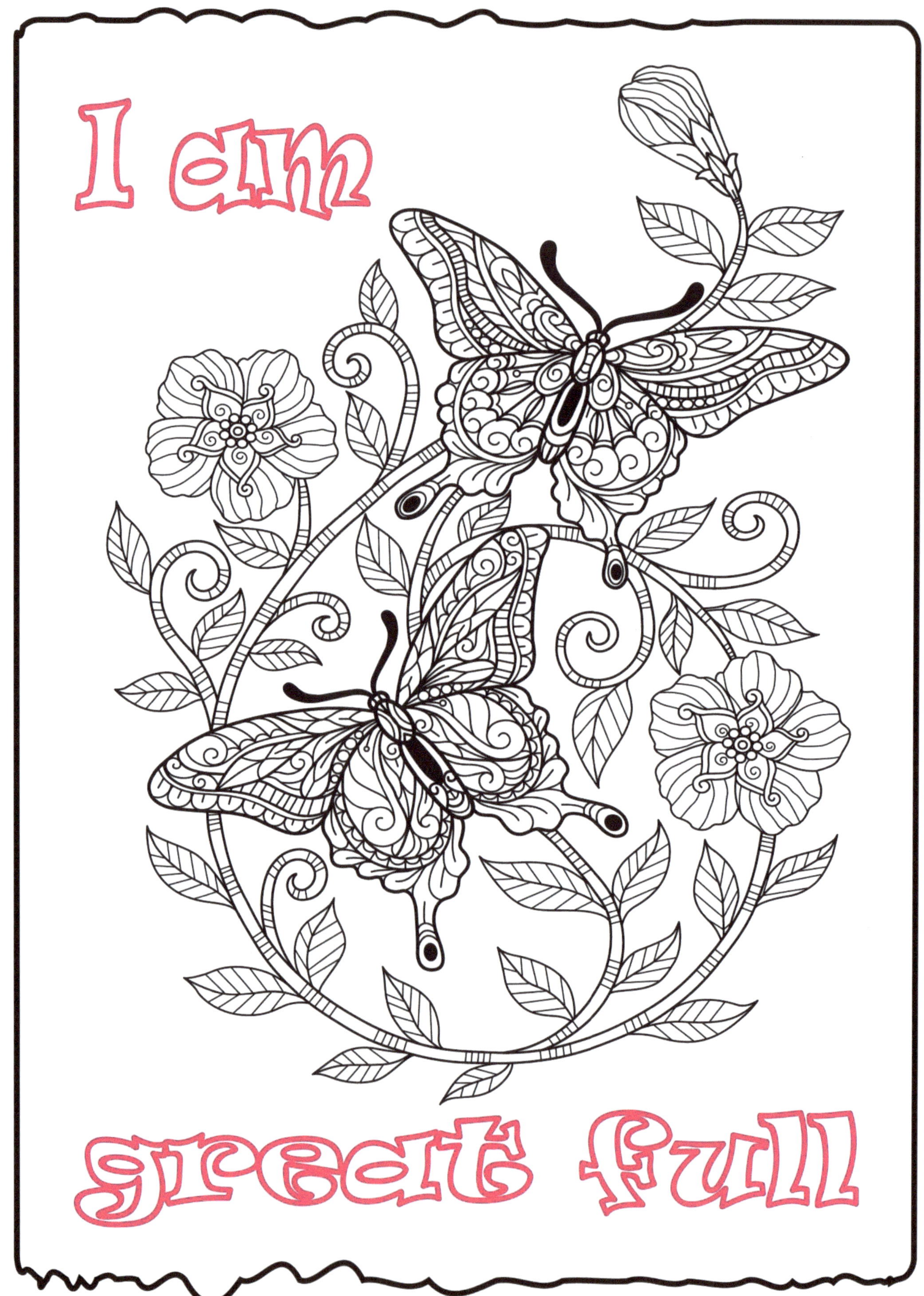
I am
great full

it's just a bad

day not a bad life

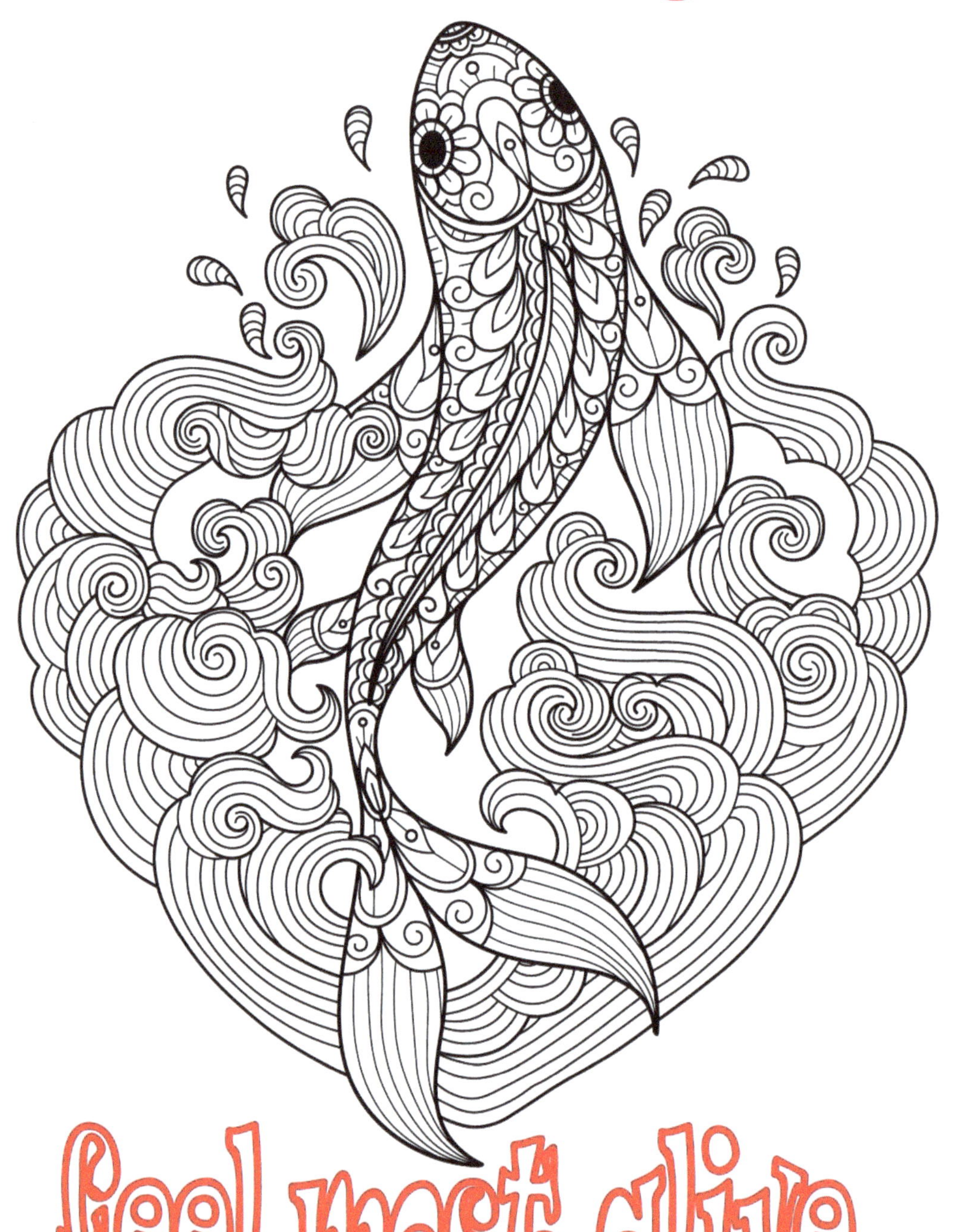
Go where you
feel most alive

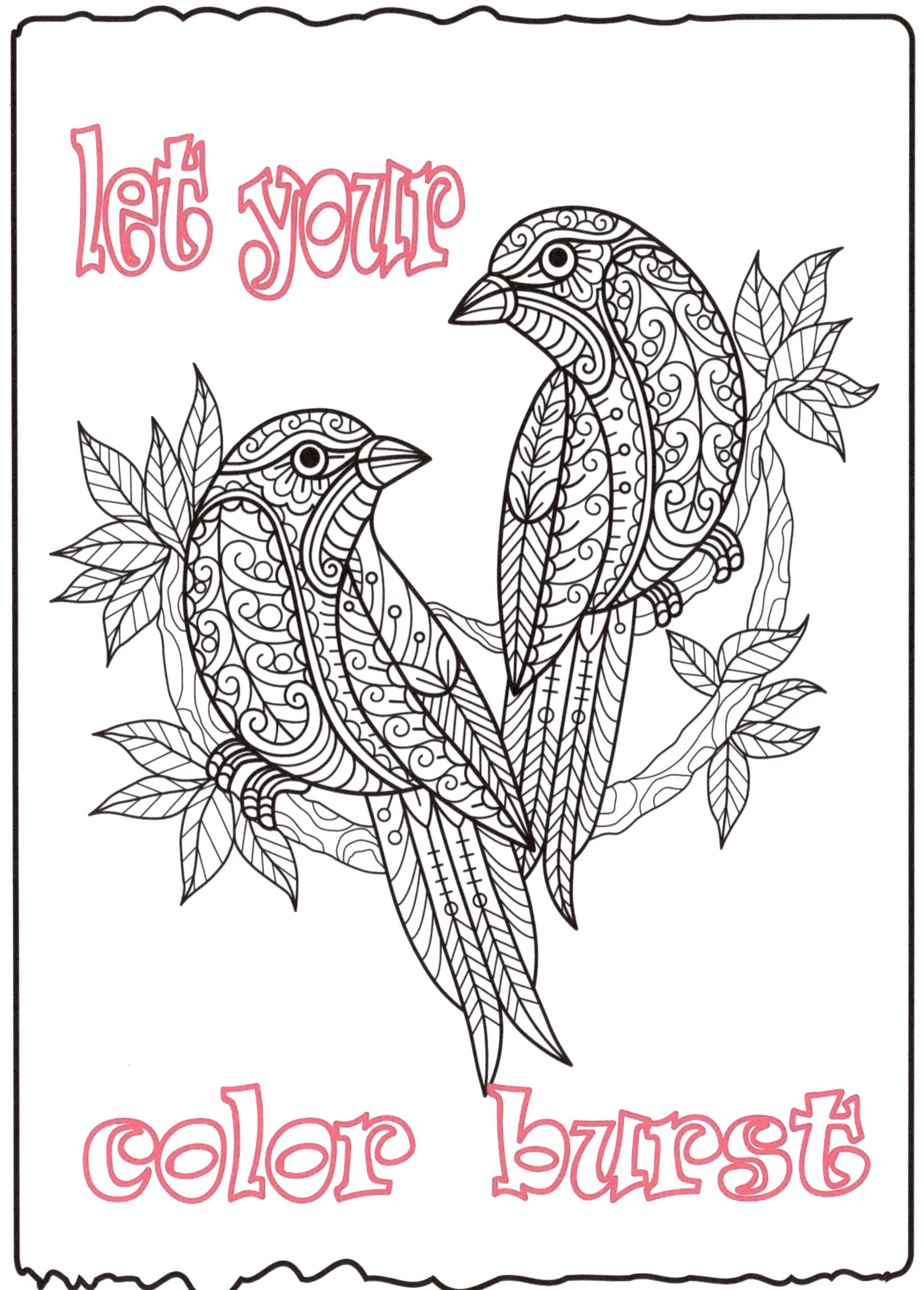

let your
color burst

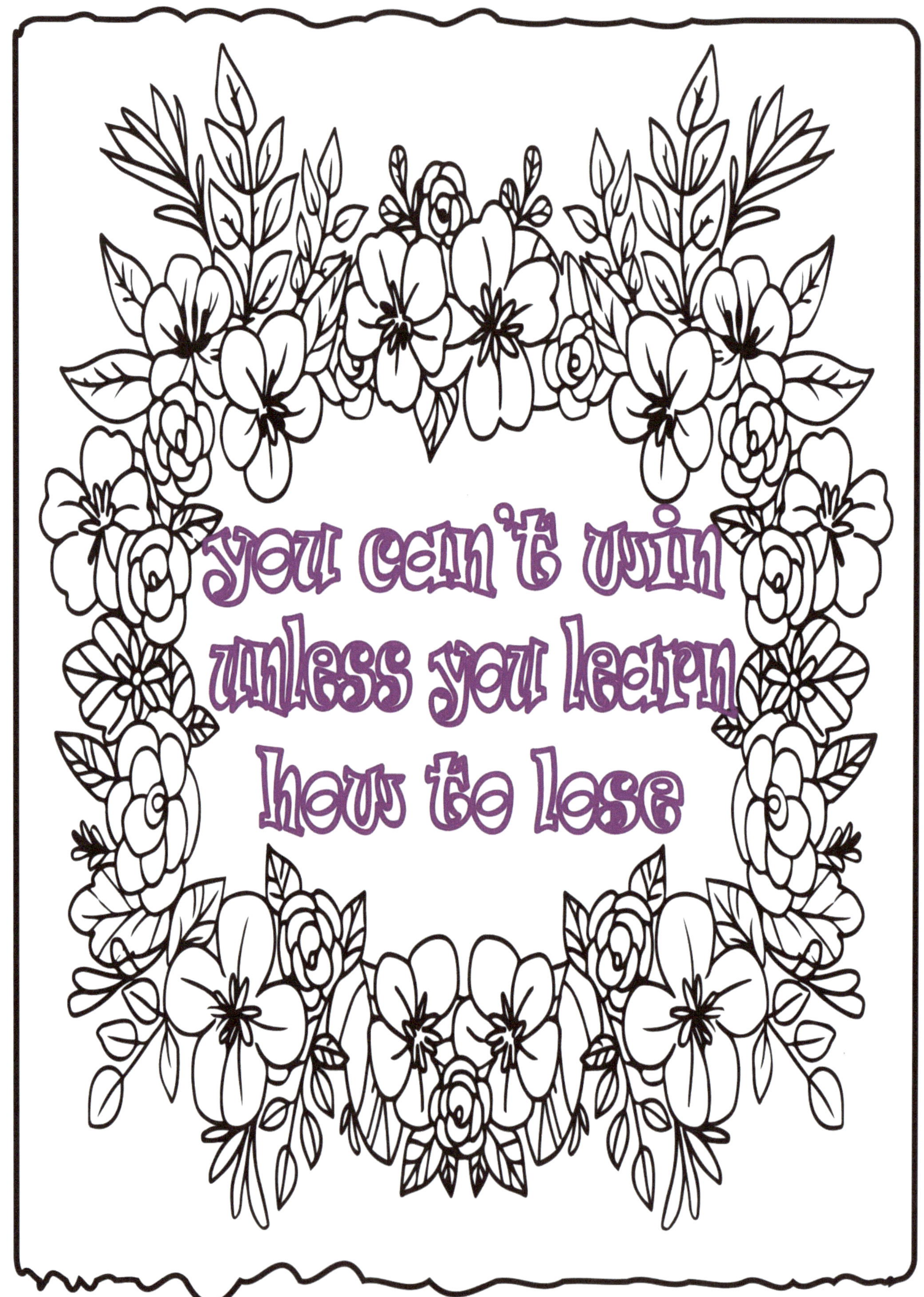

you can't win
unless you learn
how to lose

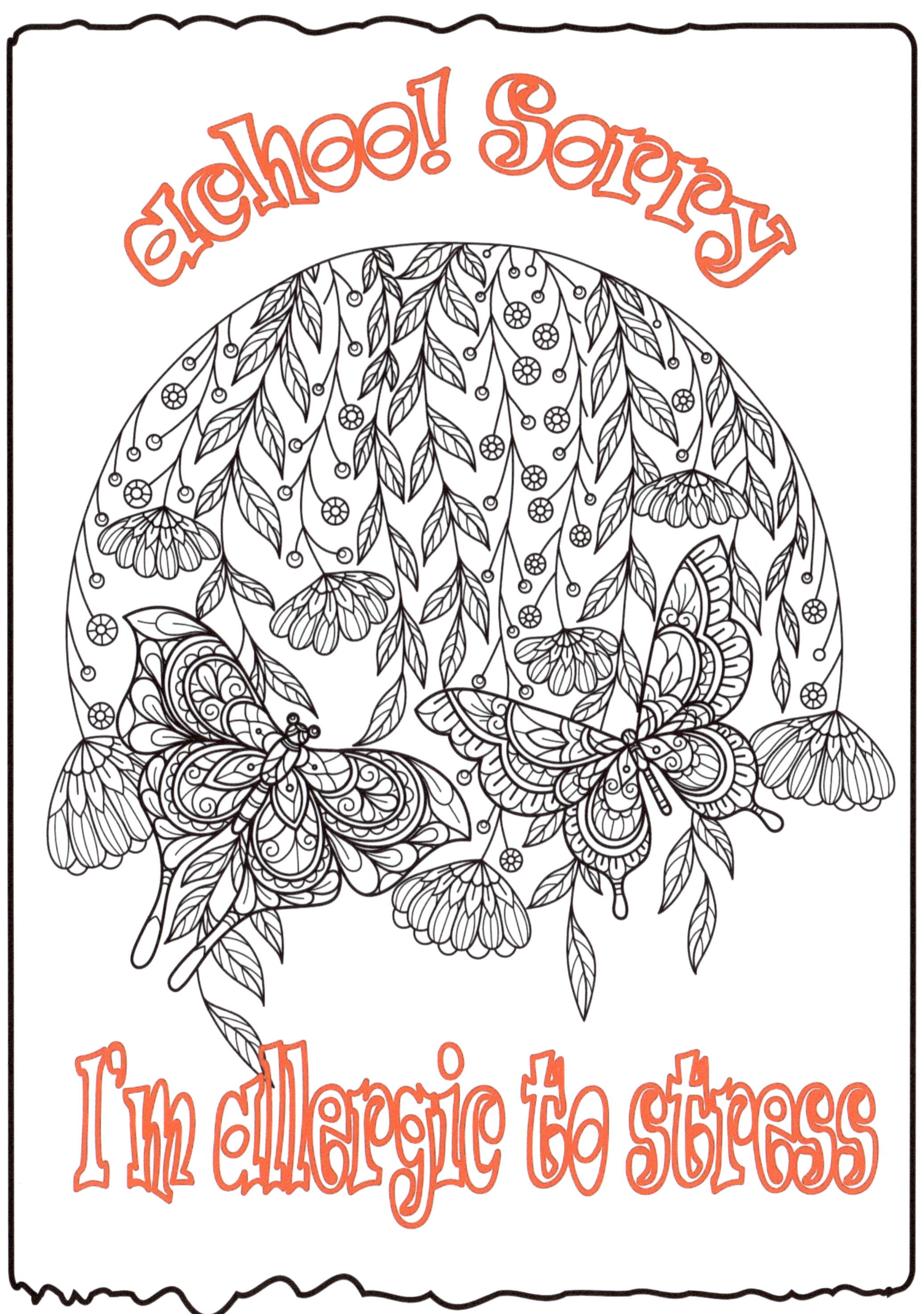

achoo! Sorry
I'm allergic to stress

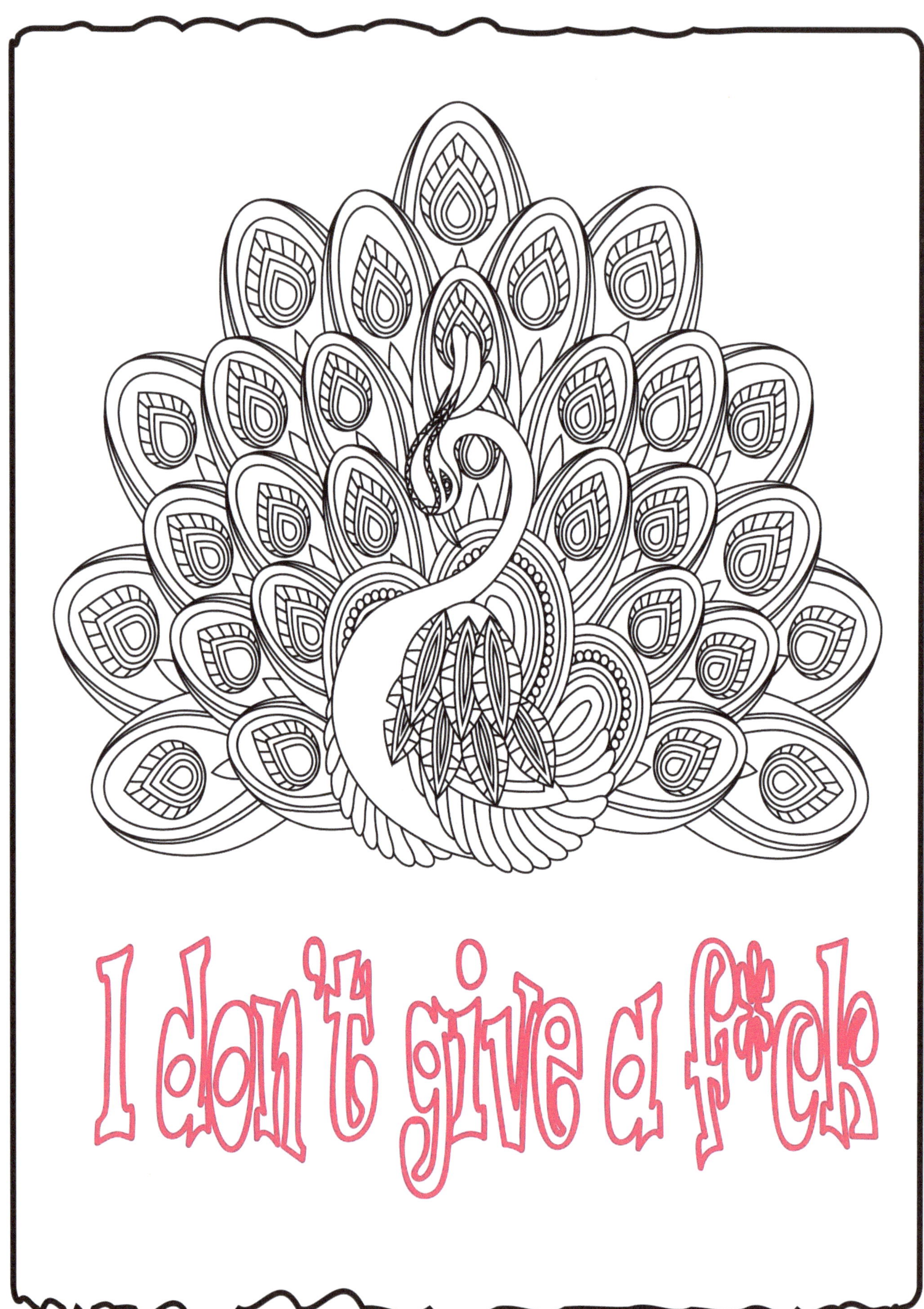
I don't give a f*ck

stress free zone

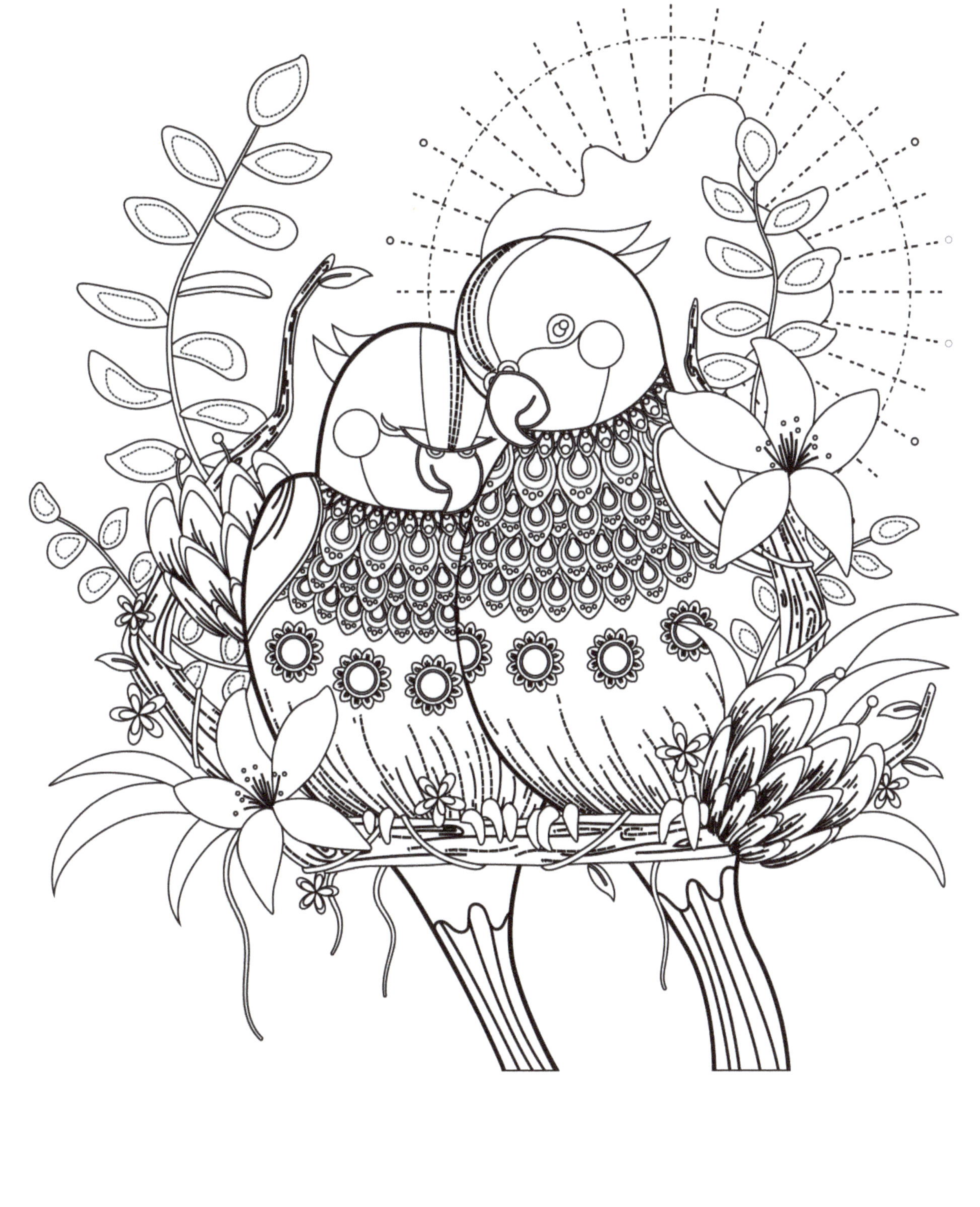

Relax we're all crazy

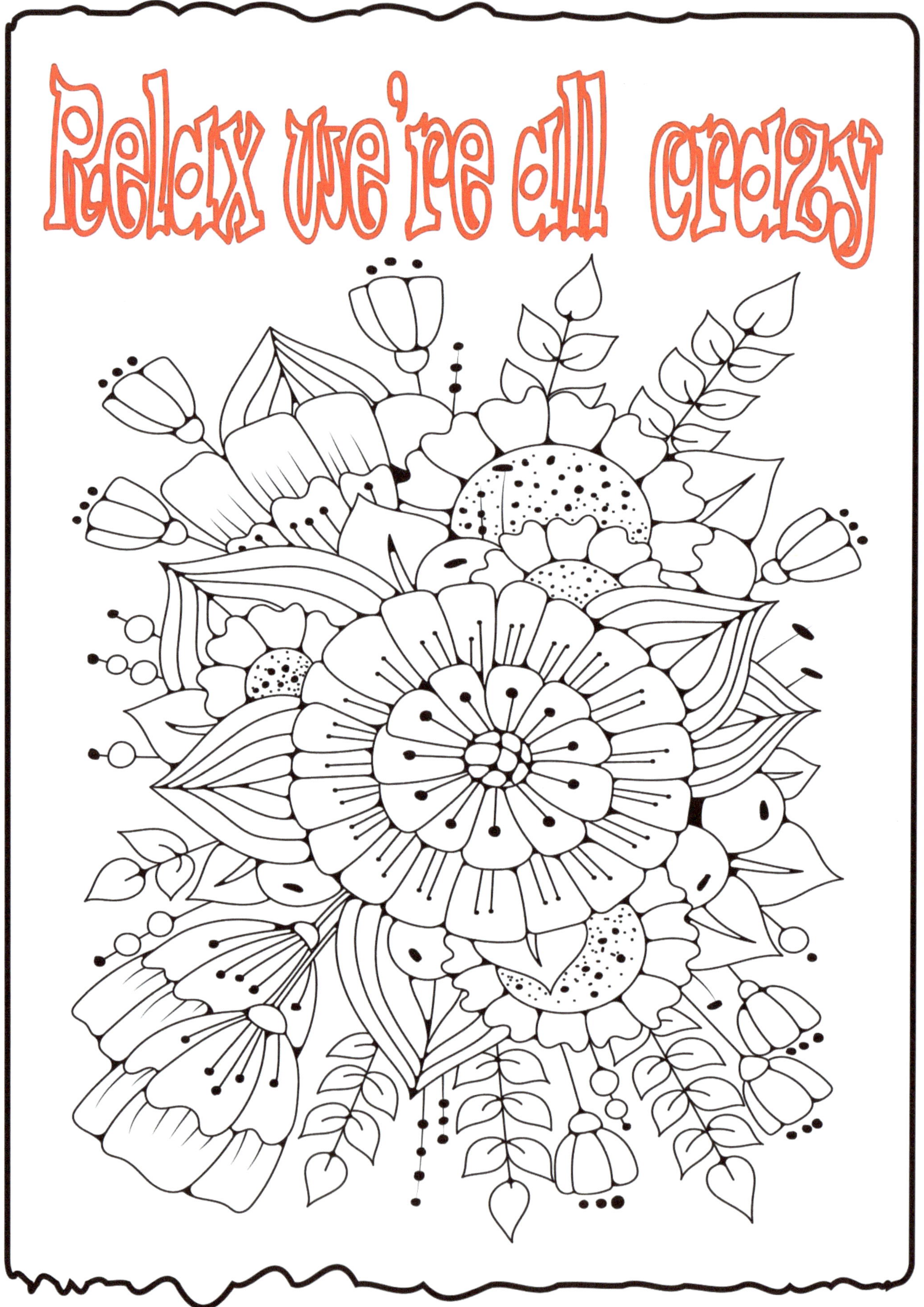

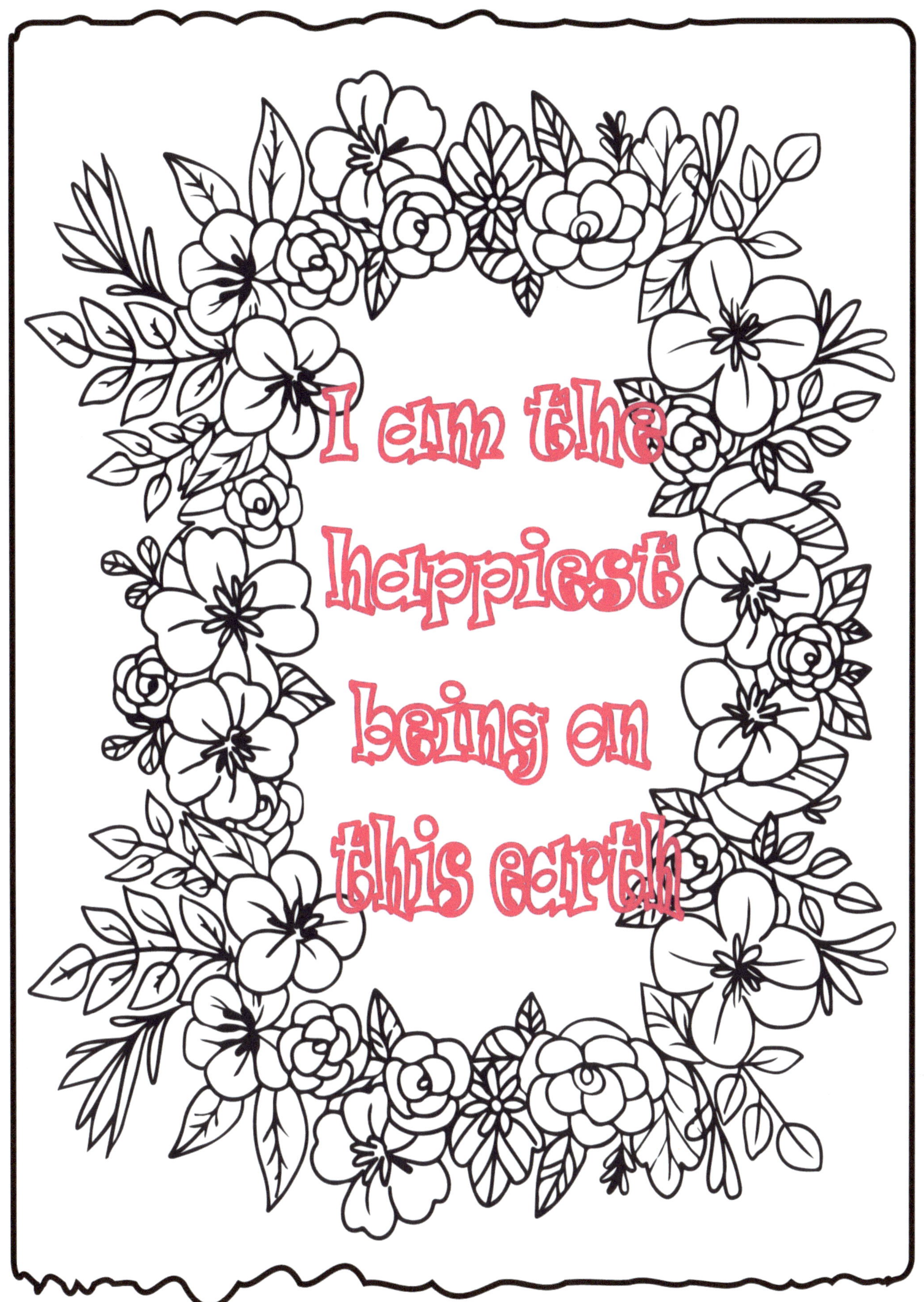

I am the
happiest
being on
this earth

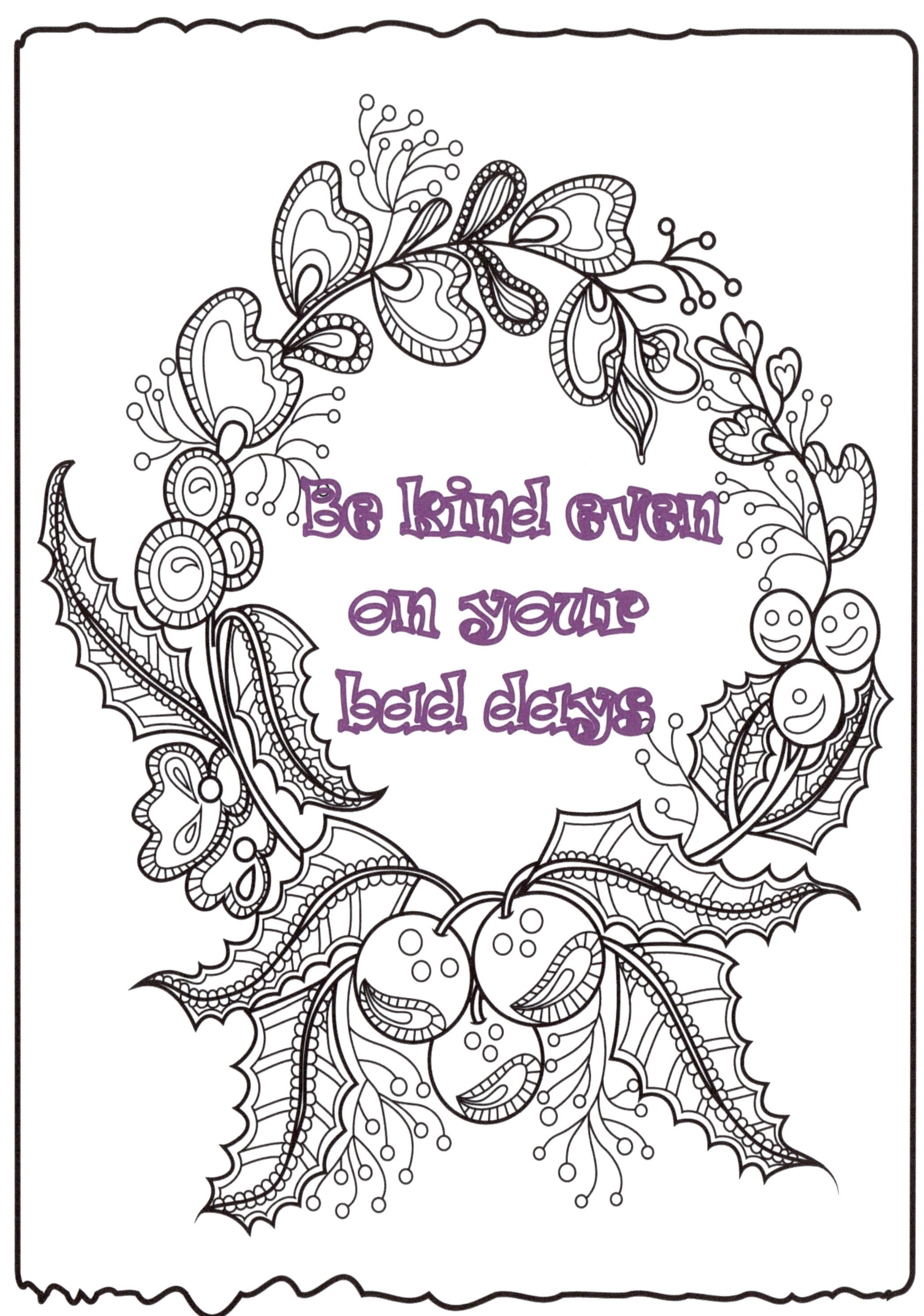
Be kind even on your bad days

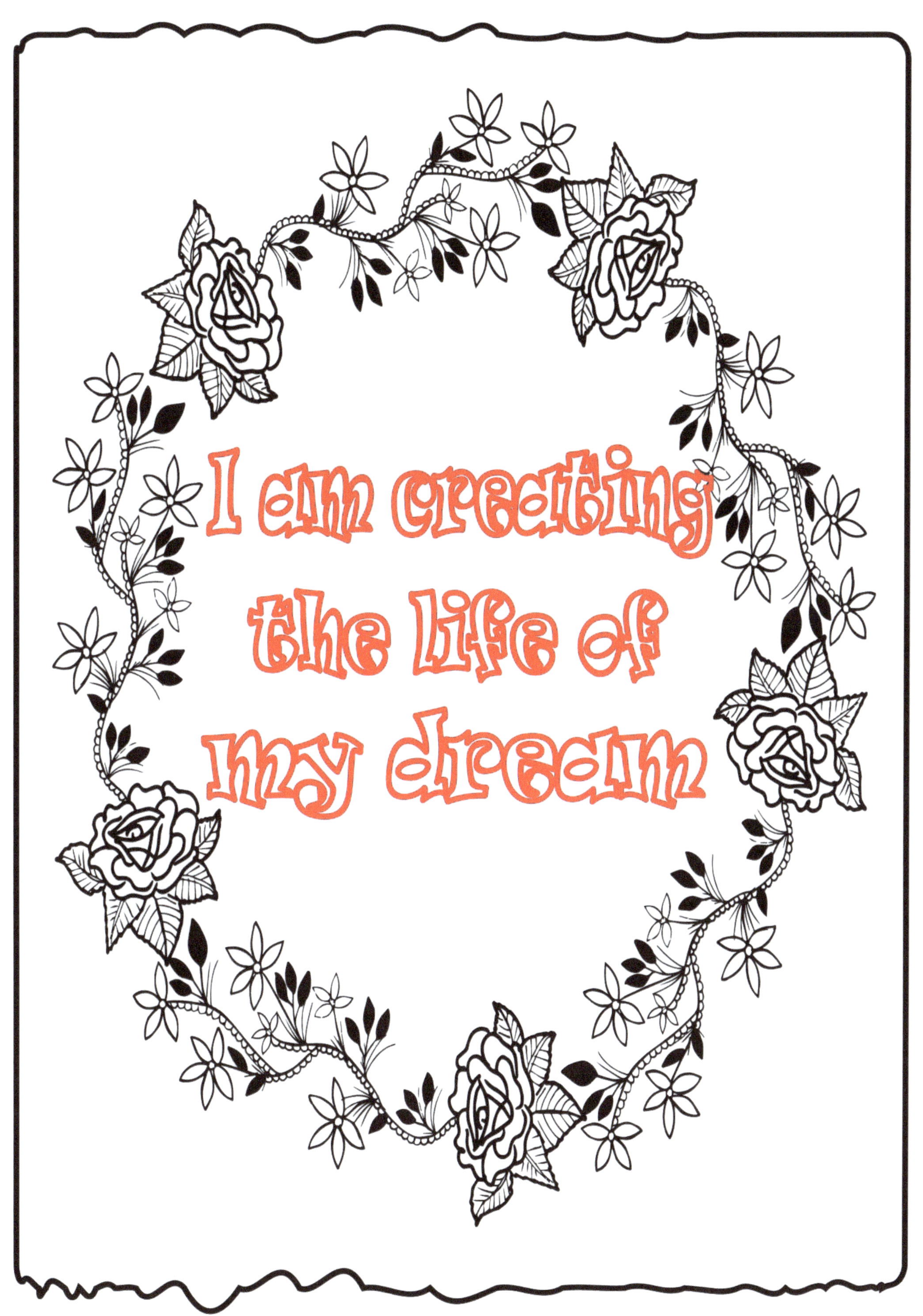

I am creating
the life of
my dream

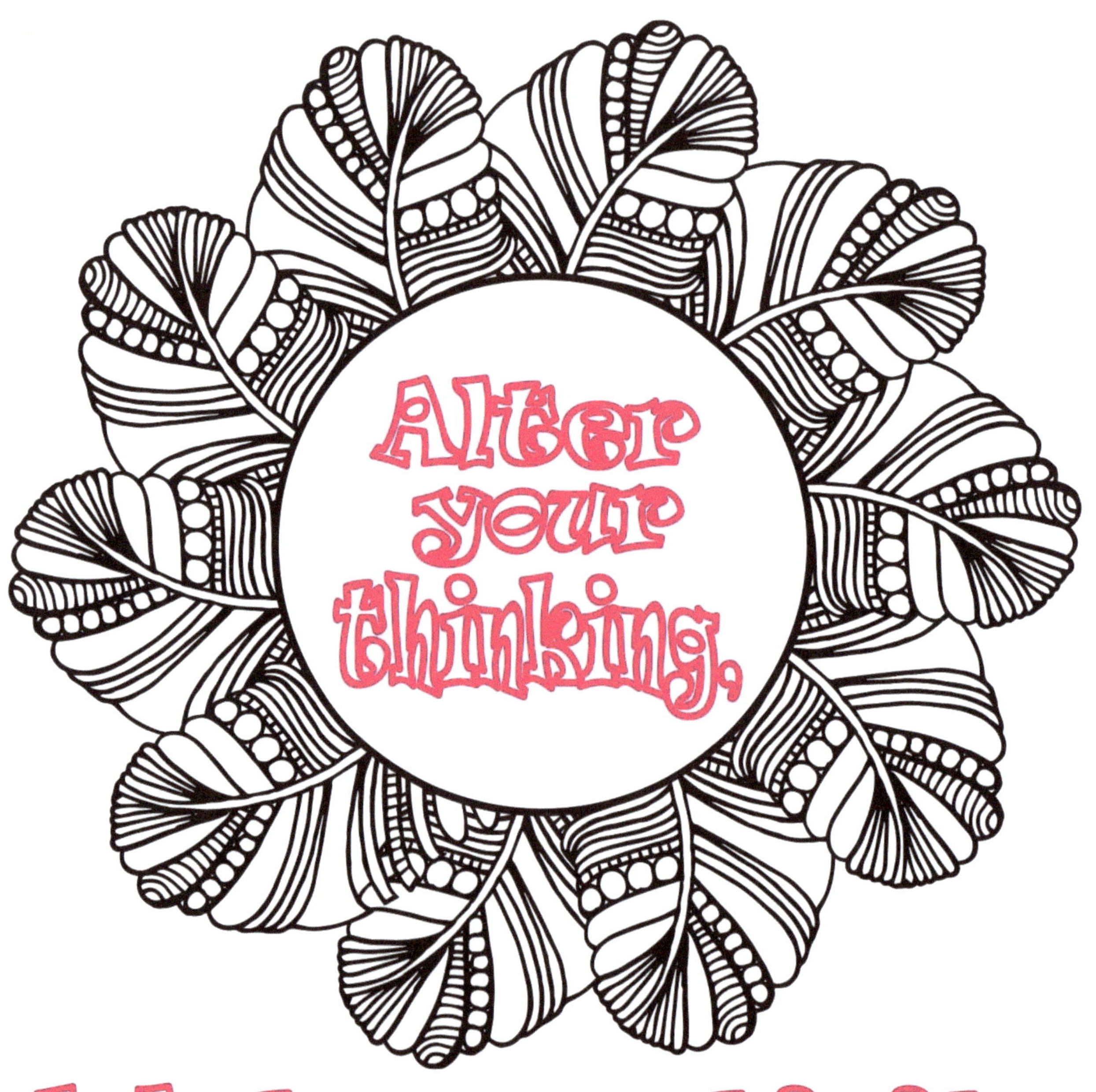

Control you self,
Alter your thinking,
delete negativity

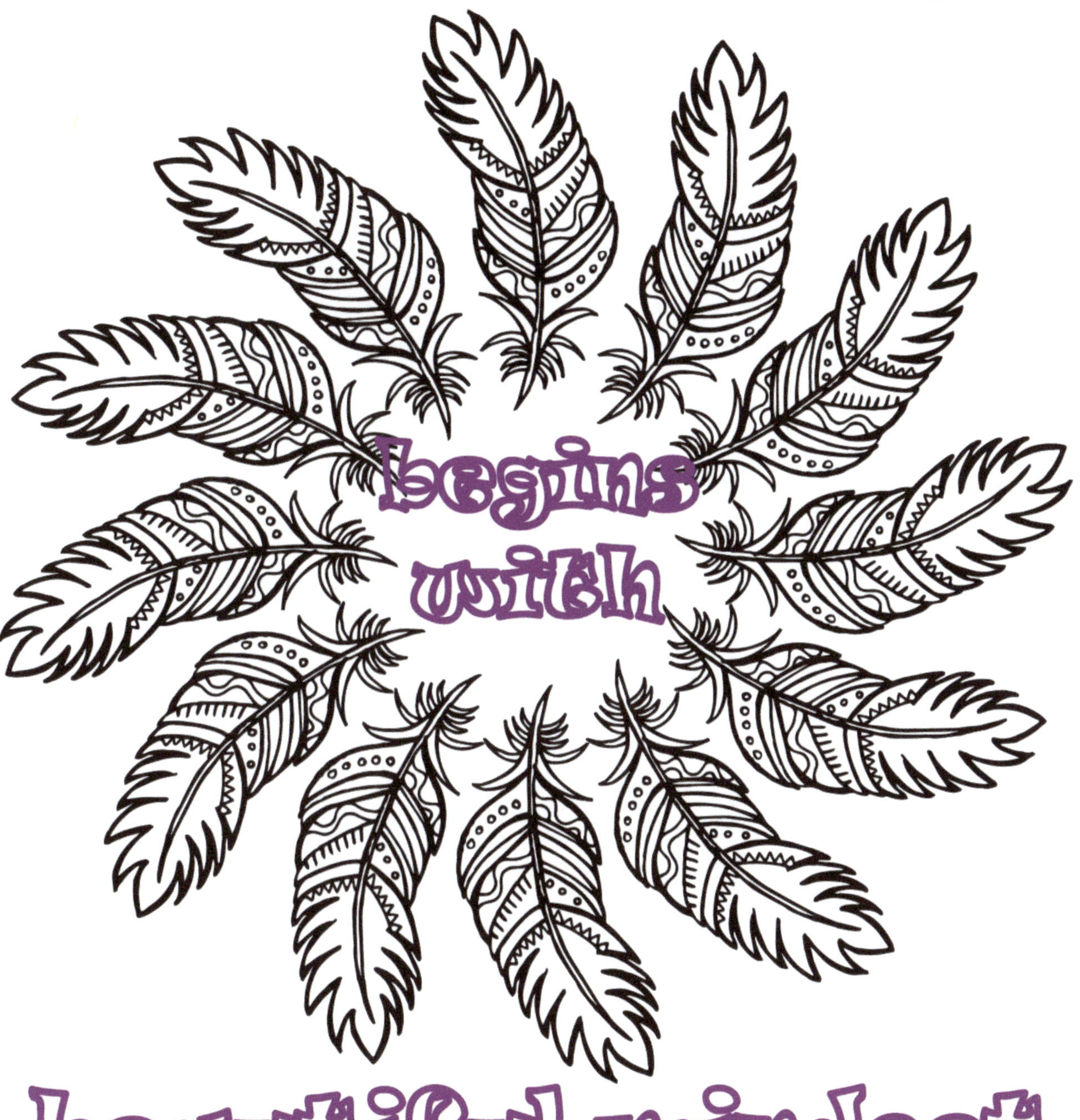

A beautiful day
begins
with
beautiful mindset

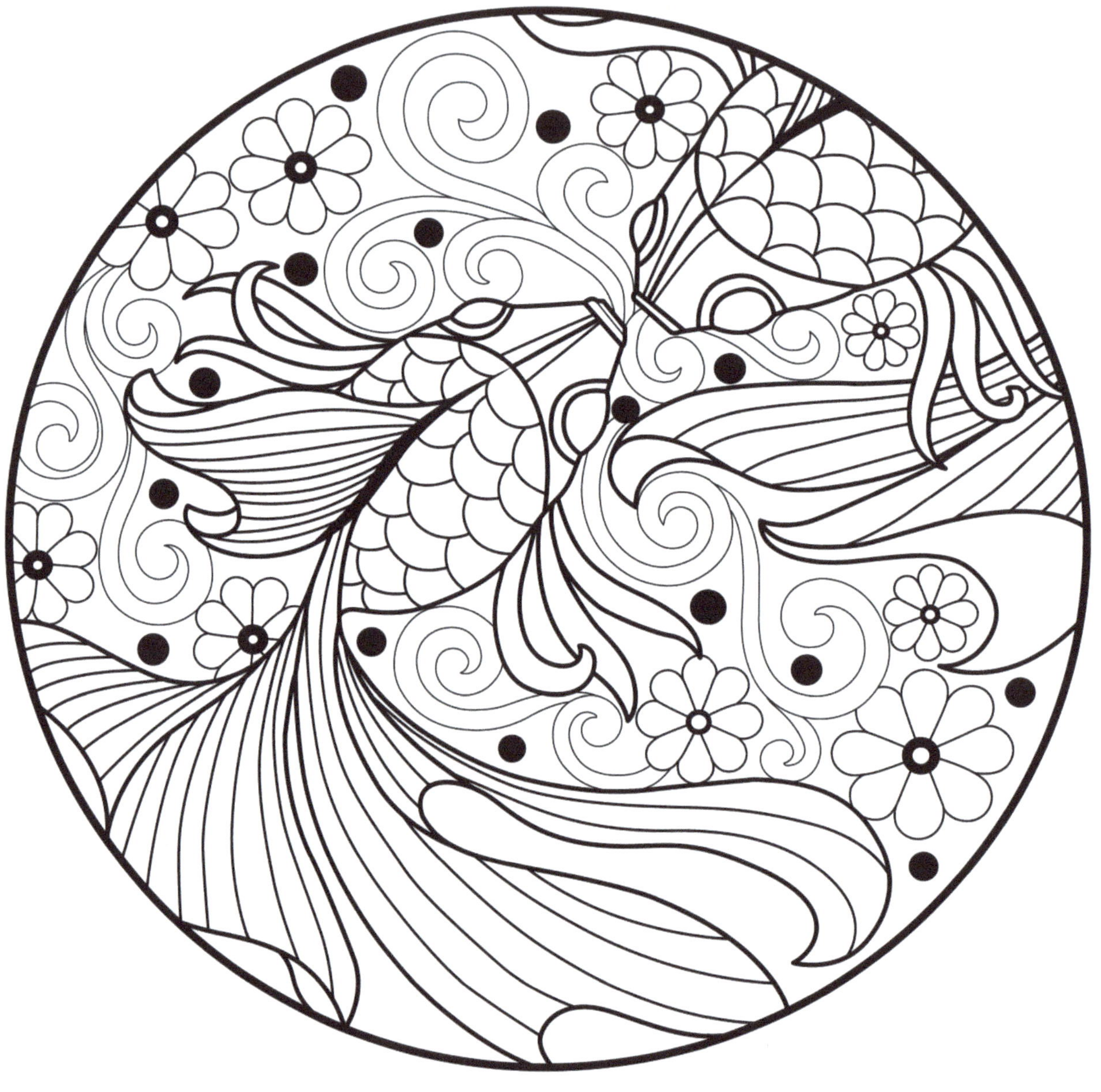
your only limit
is your mind

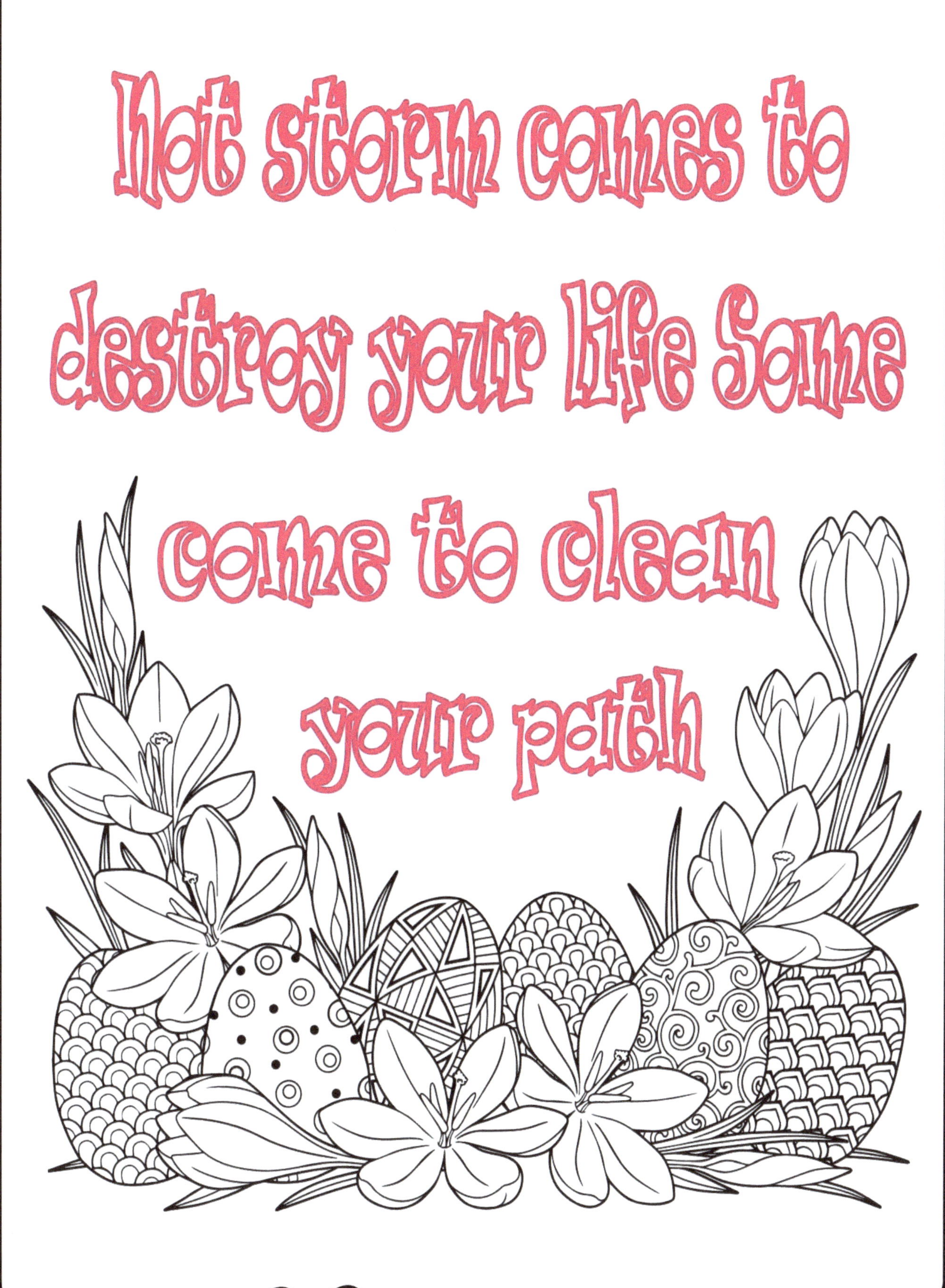

not storm comes to destroy your life Some come to clean your path

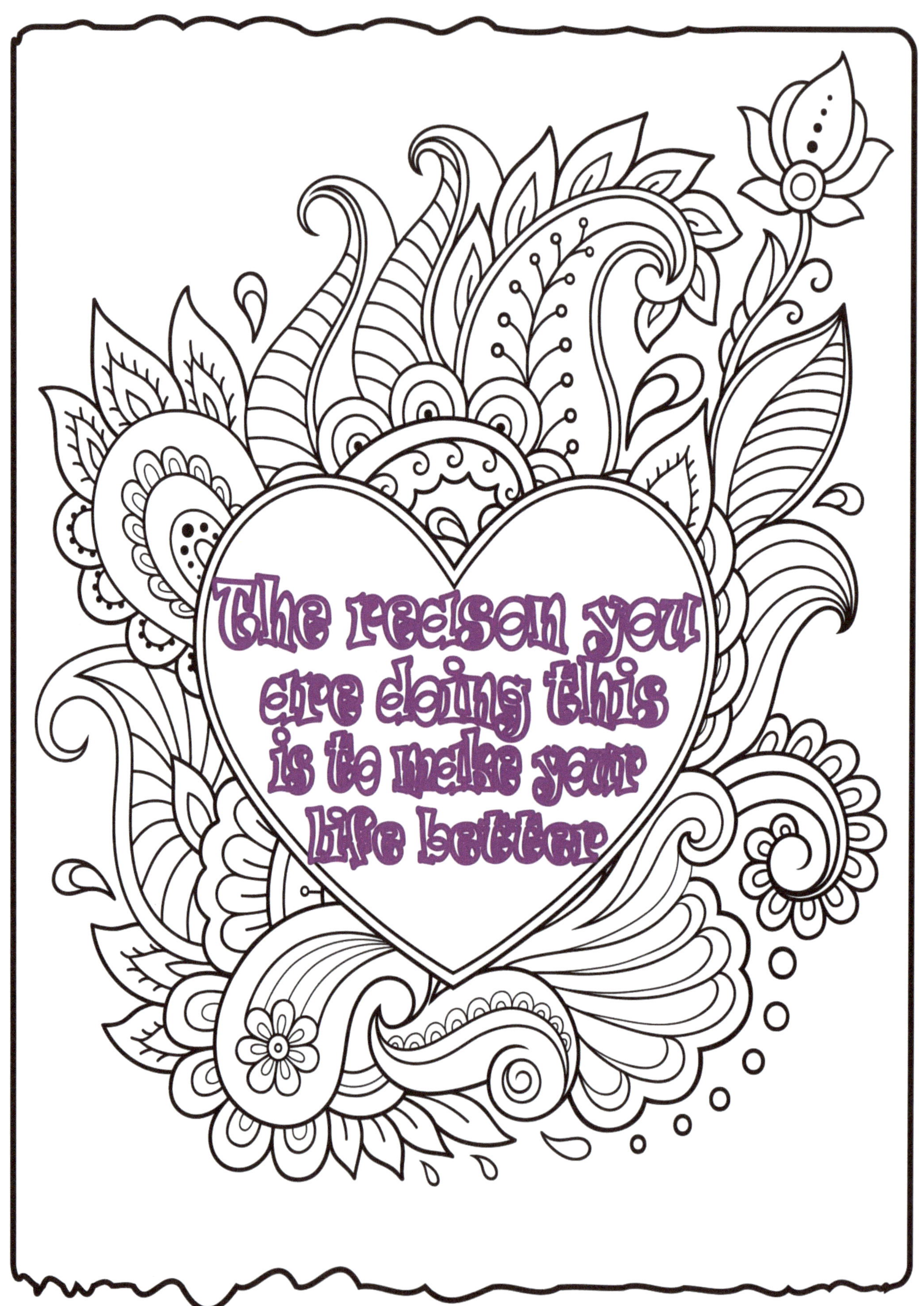

The reason you
are doing this
is to make your
life better

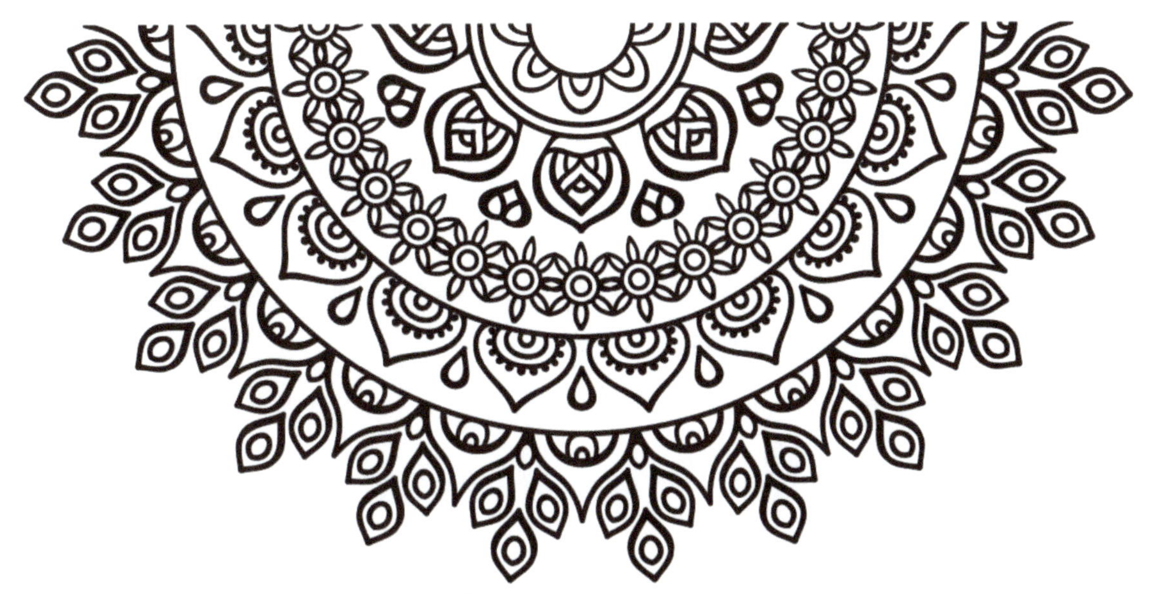

A negative mind will not give you a positive life

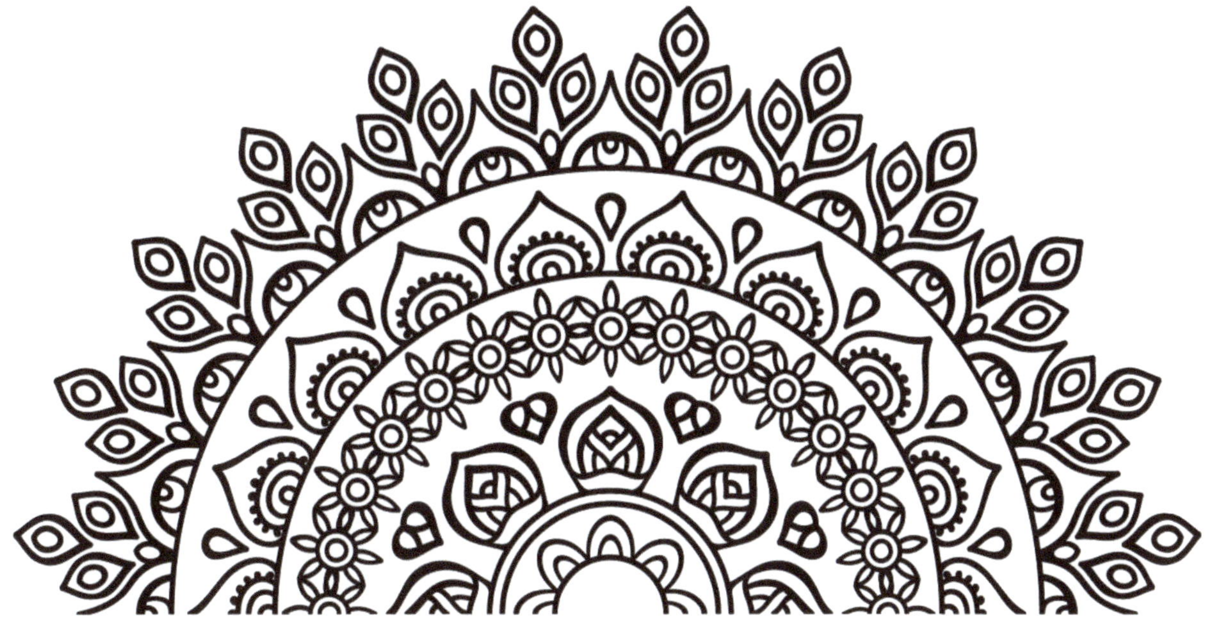

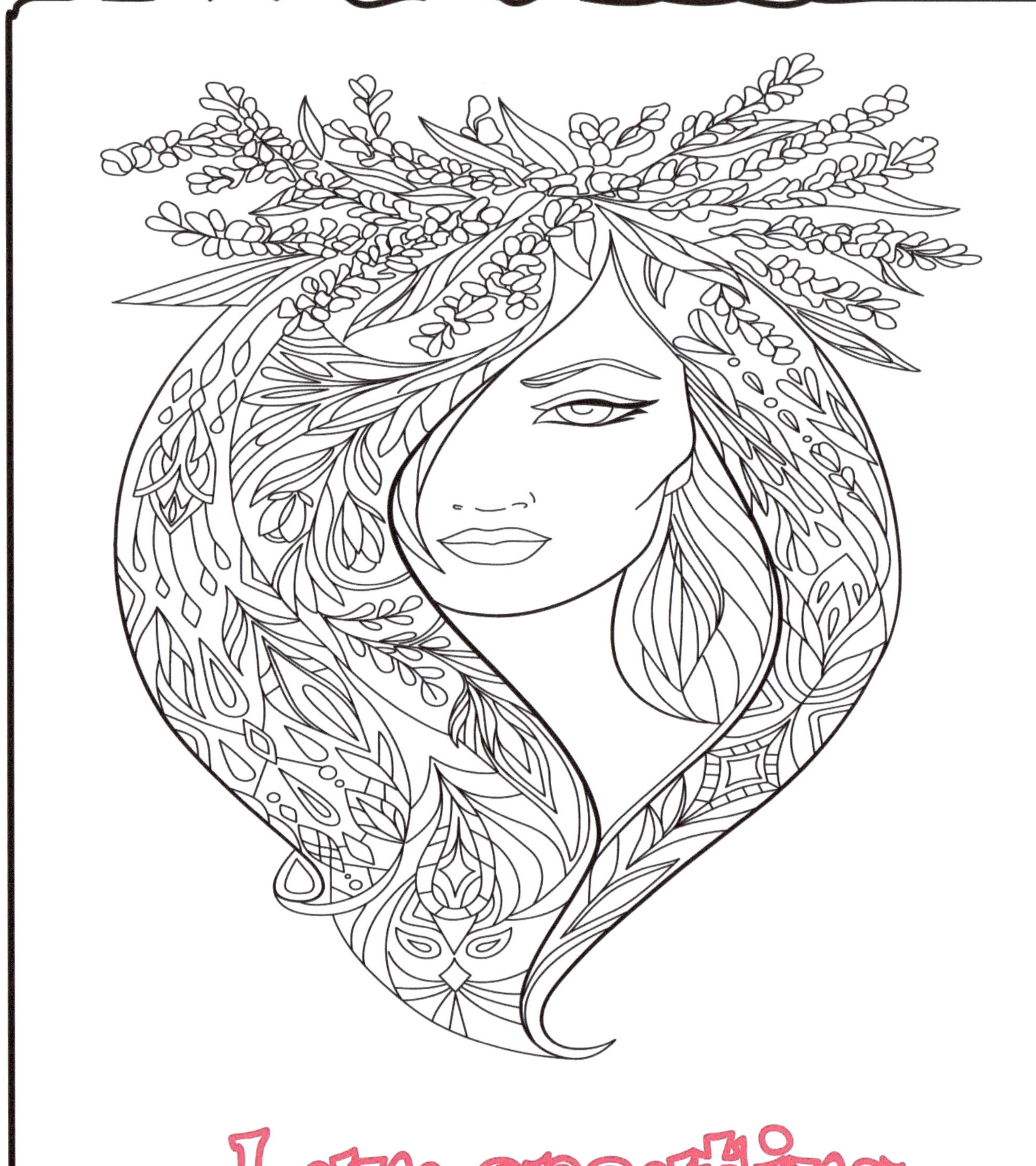

I am creating
the life of my dream

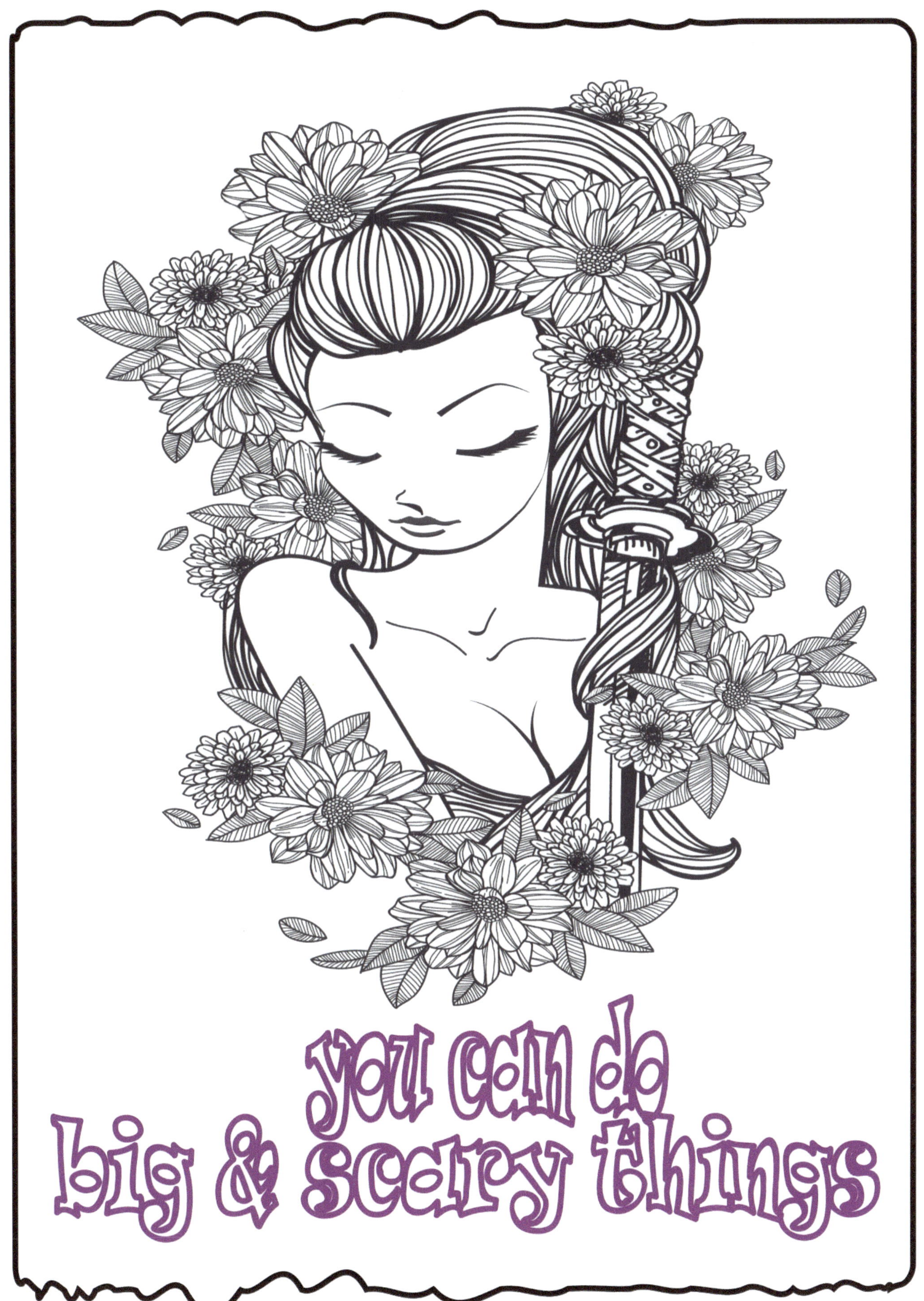

you can do
big & scary things

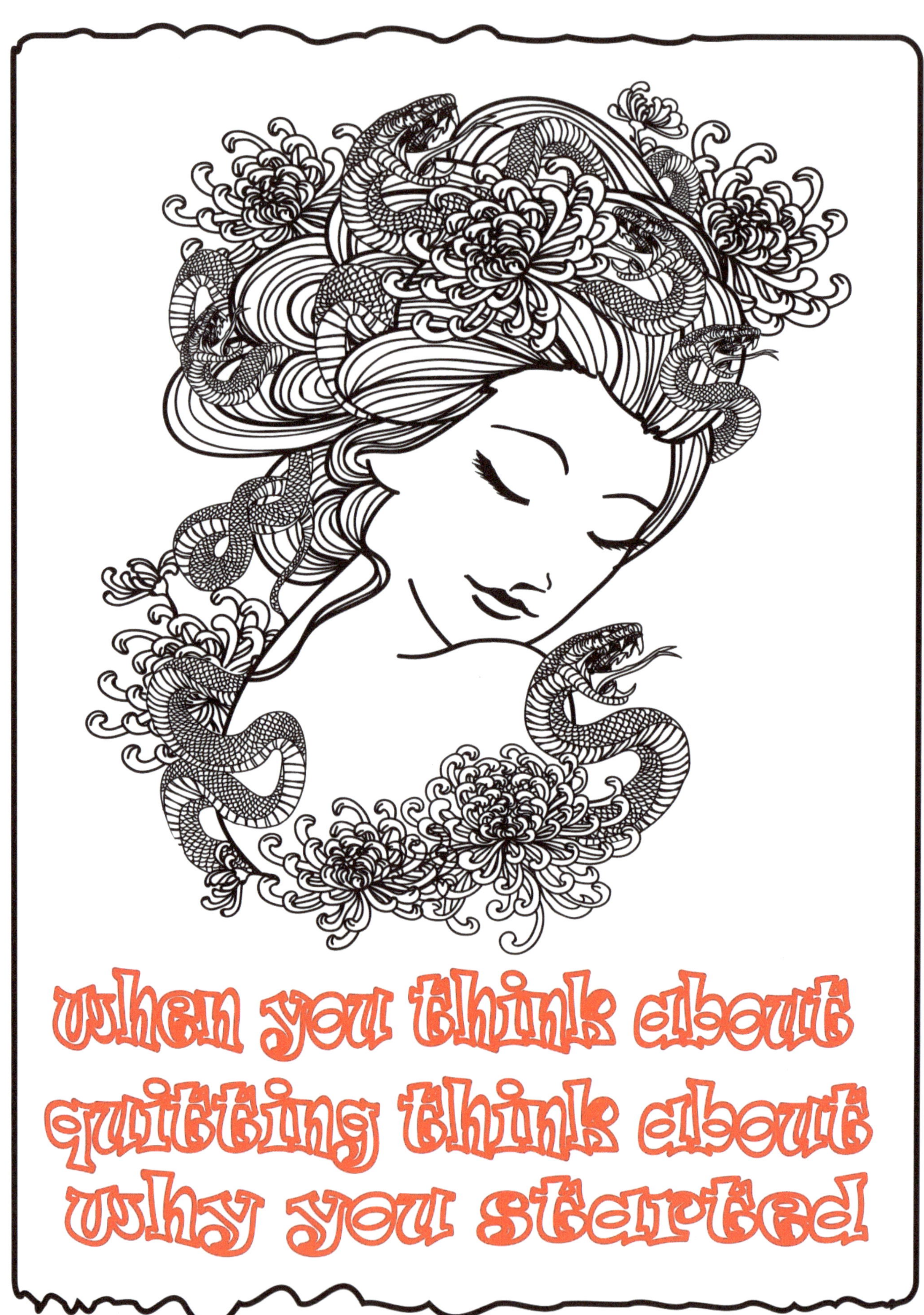
when you think about
quitting think about
why you started

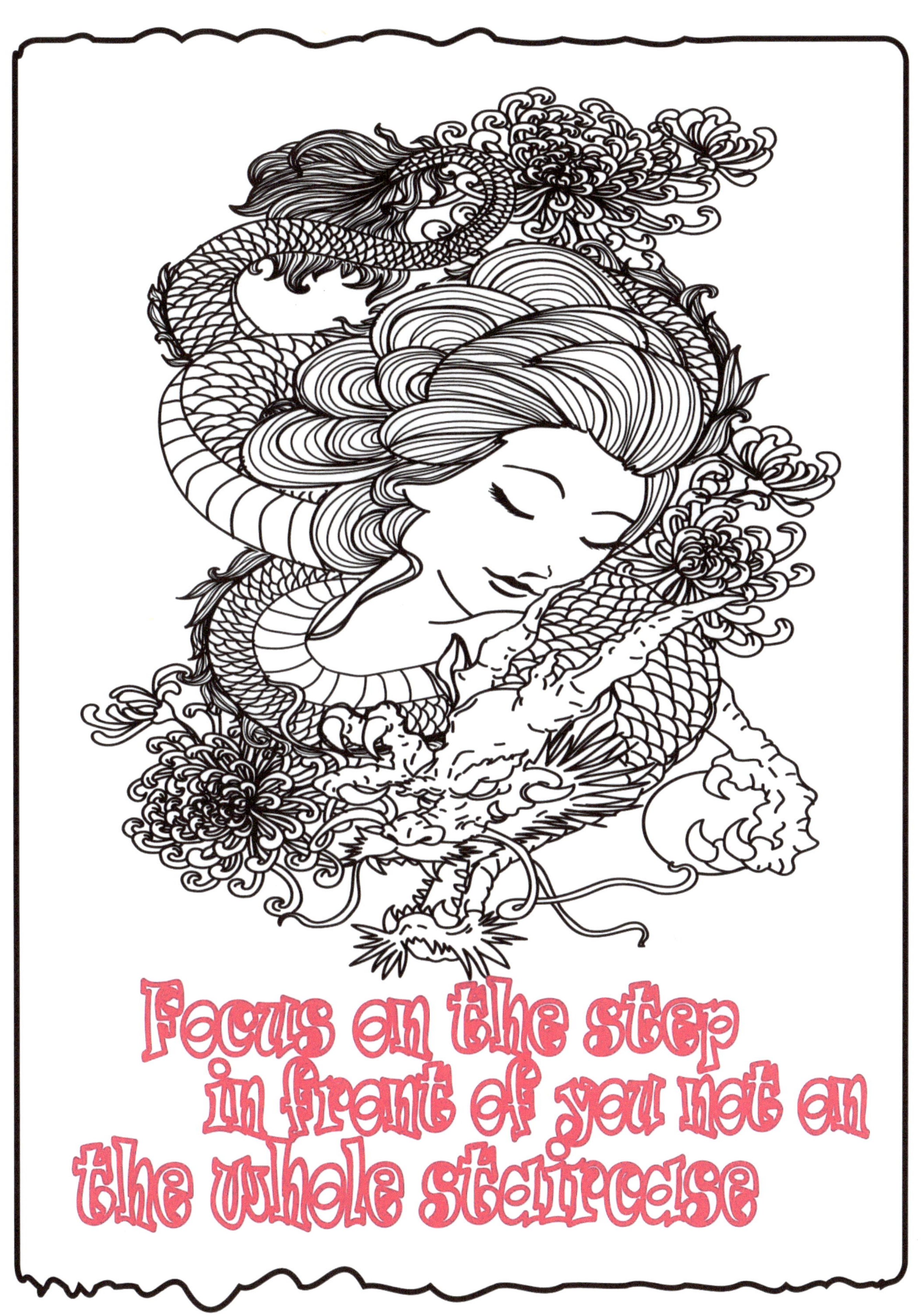
Focus on the step
in front of you not on
the whole staircase

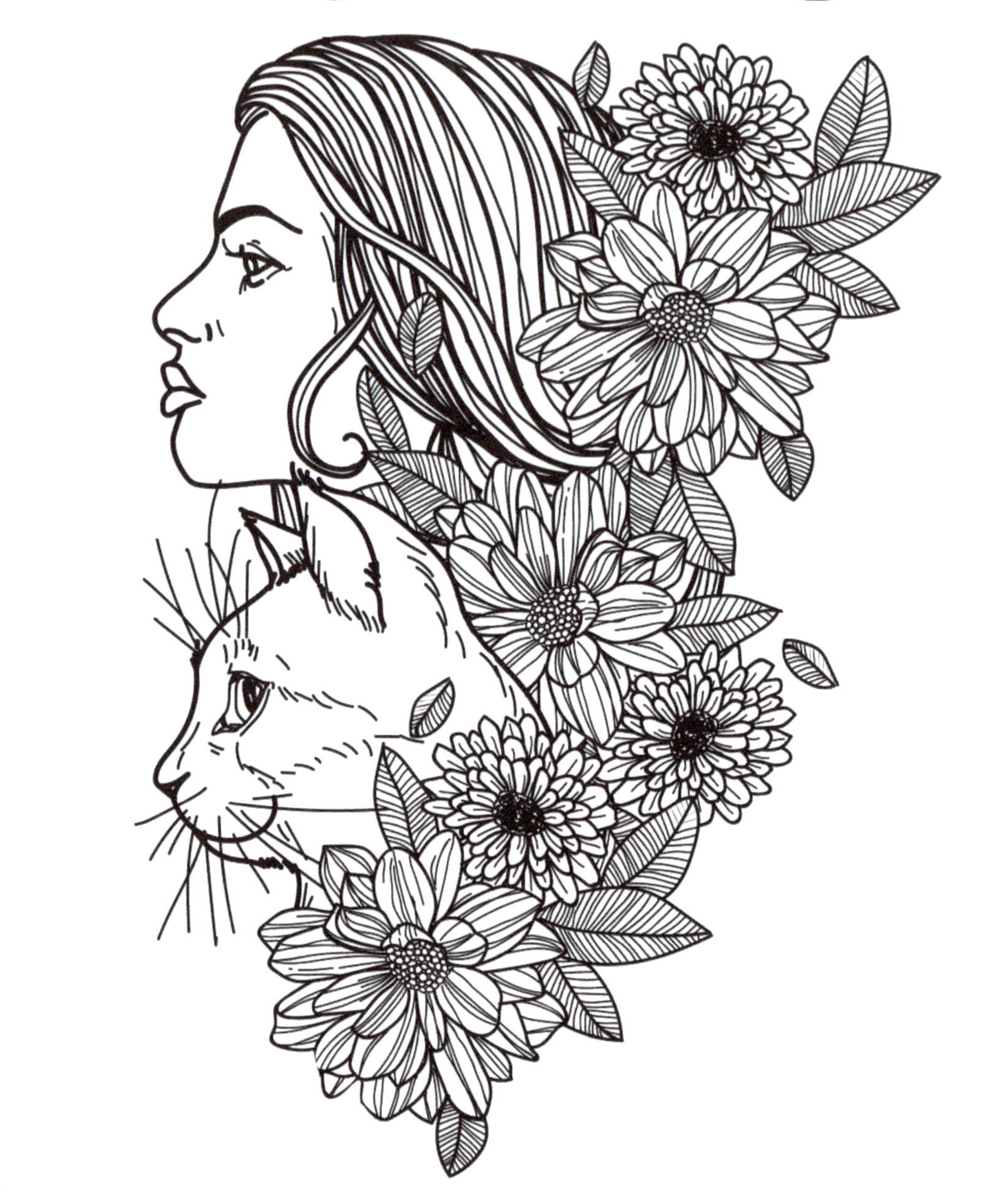

celebrate every win,
no matter how small

Train your mind to see the good in every situation

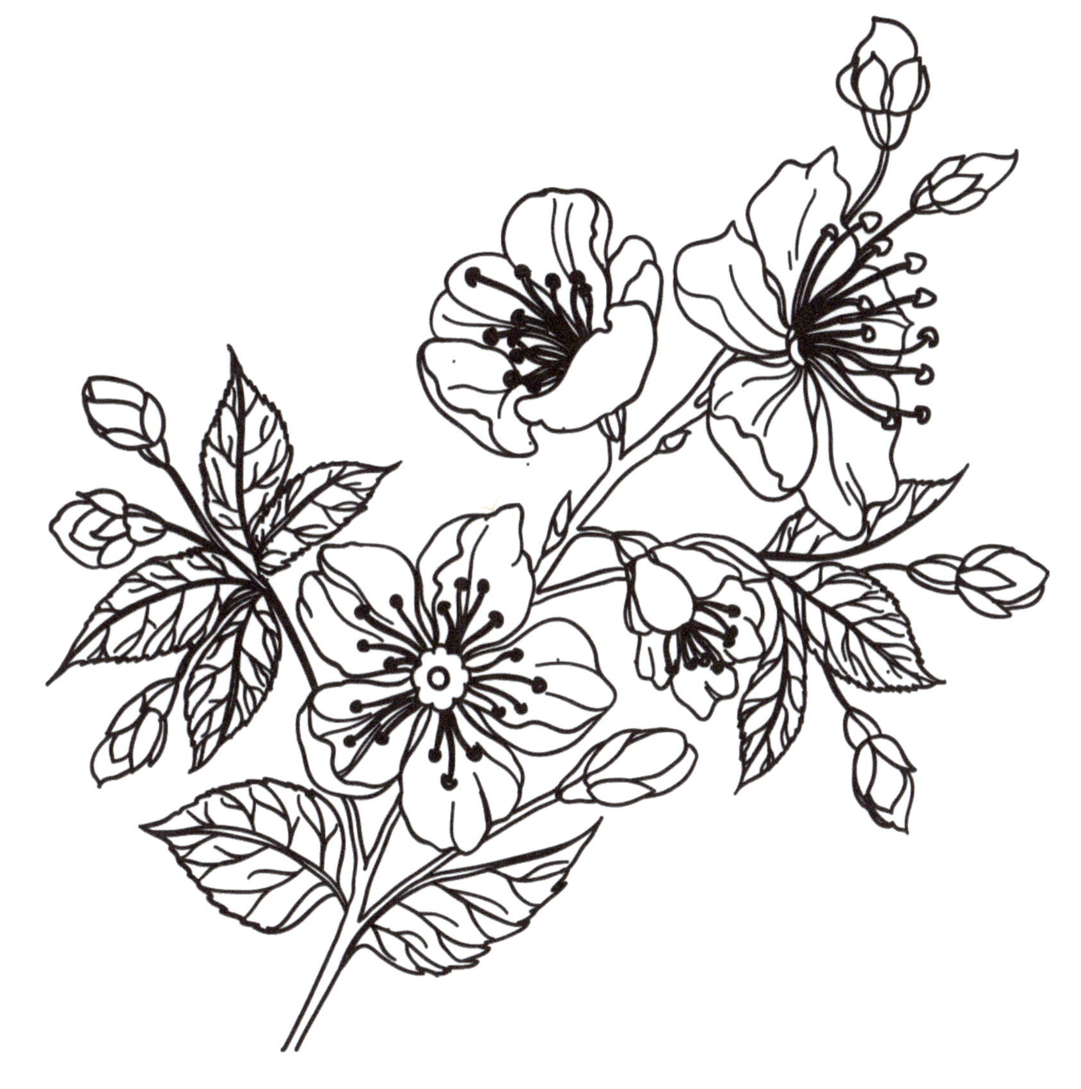

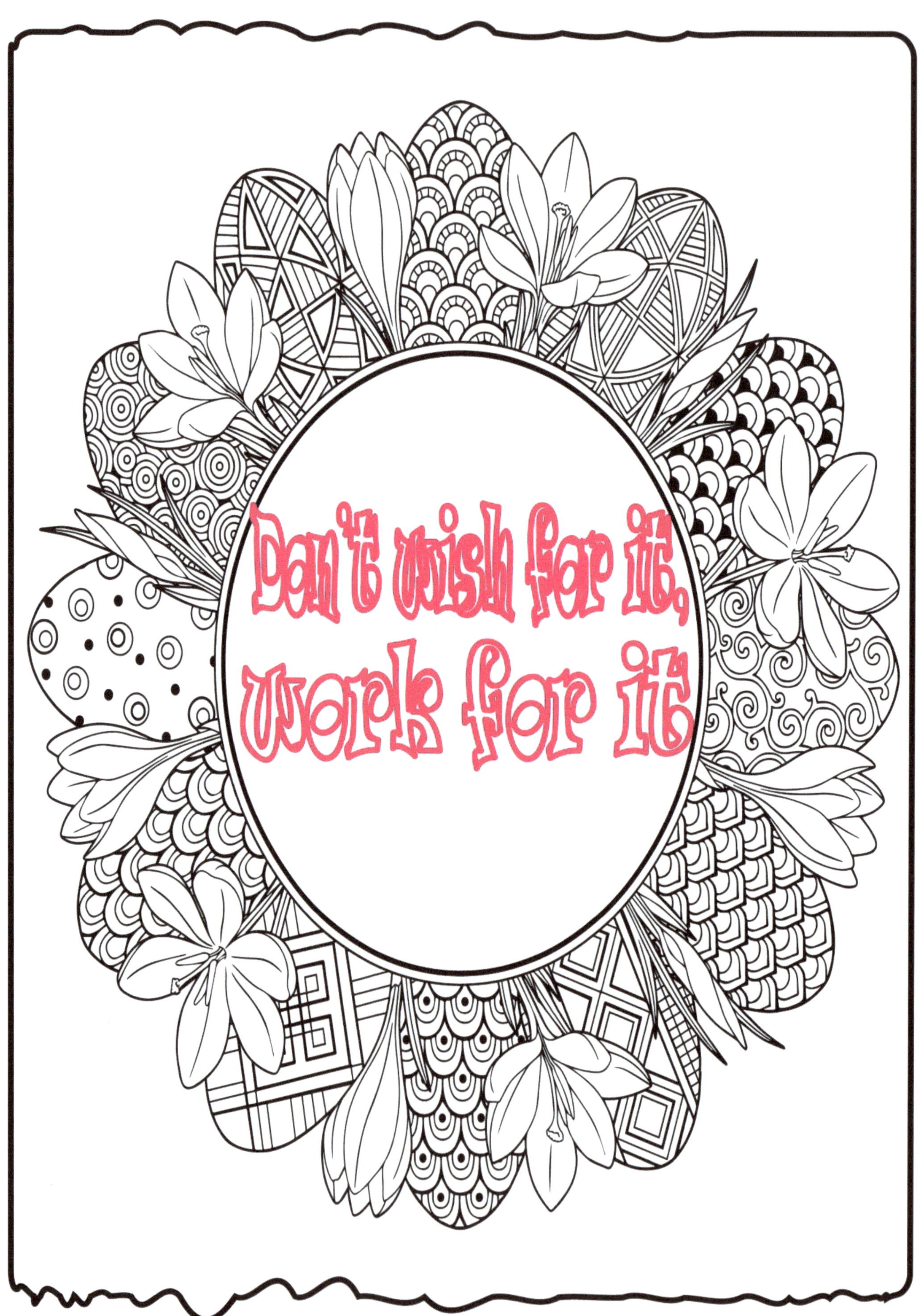
Don't wish for it,
work for it

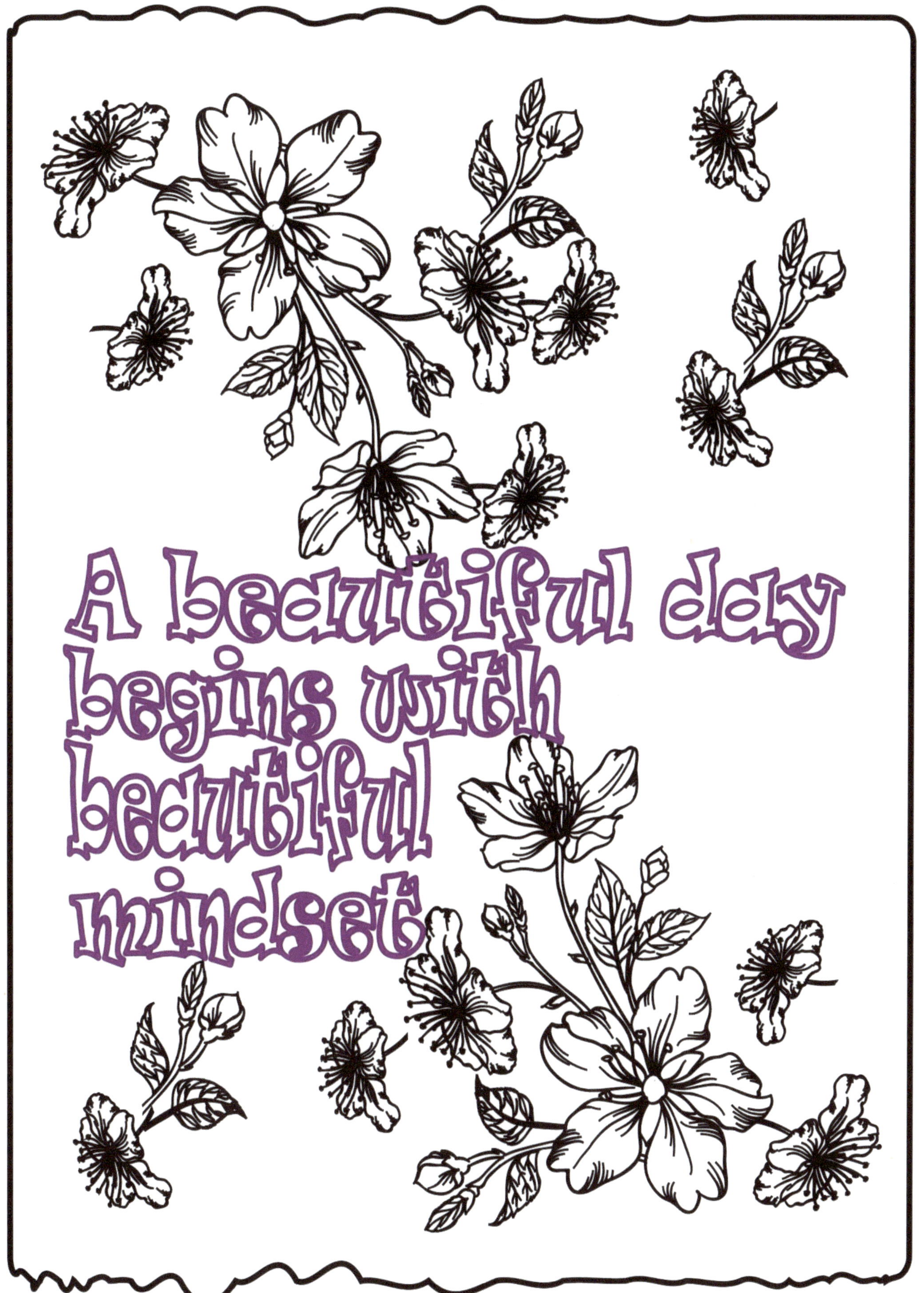

A beautiful day begins with beautiful mindset

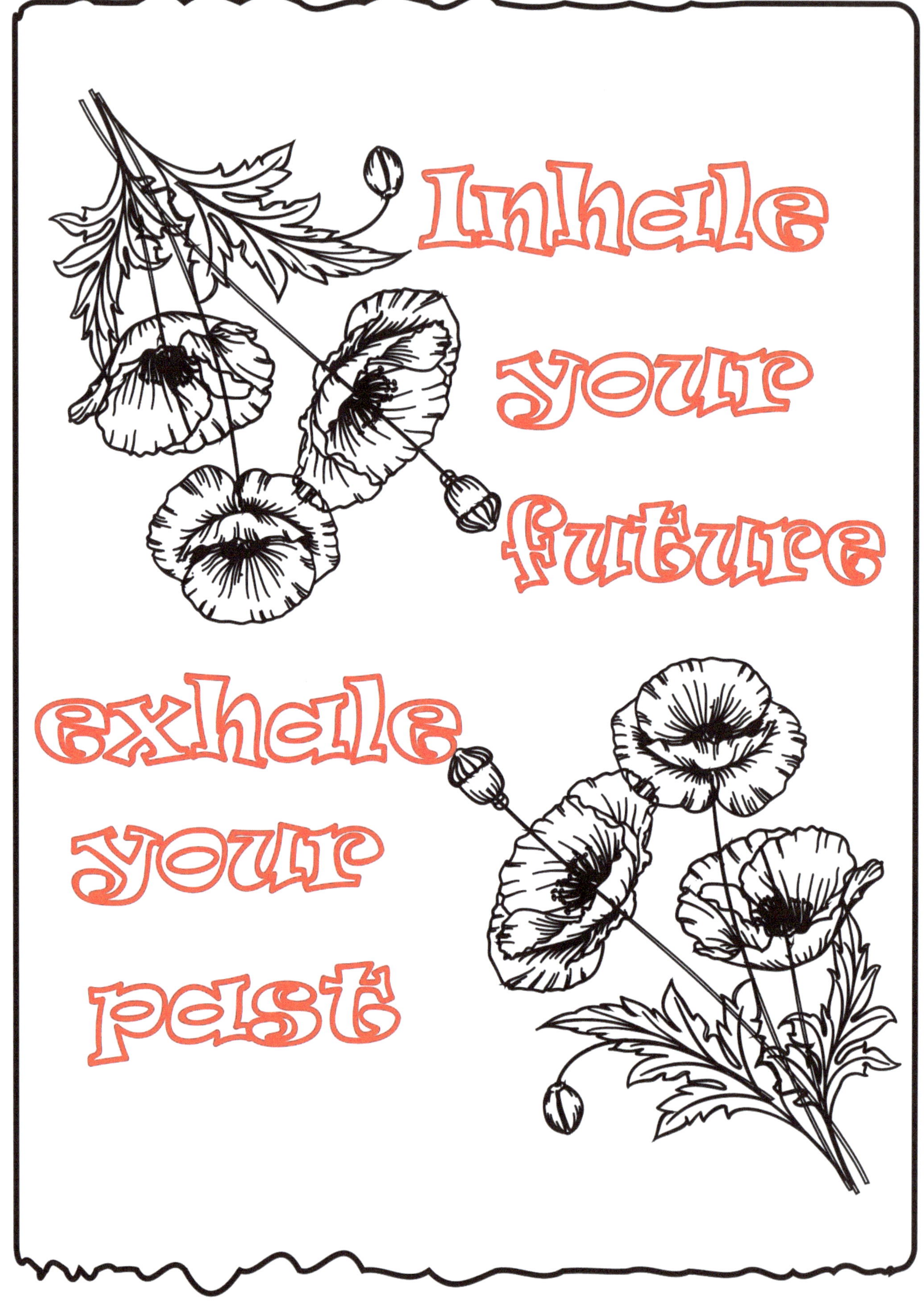

Inhale
your
future
exhale
your
past

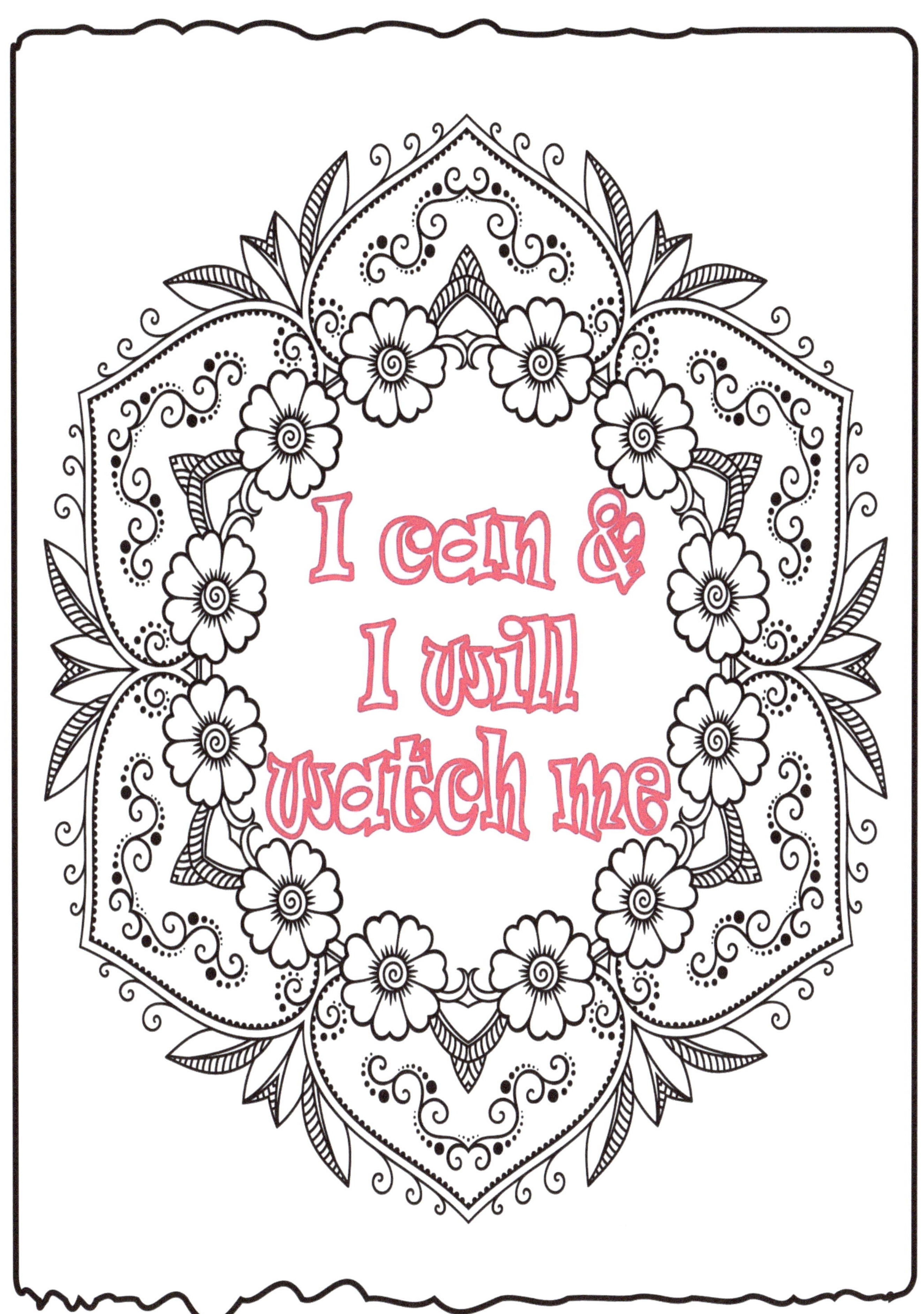

I can &
I will
watch me

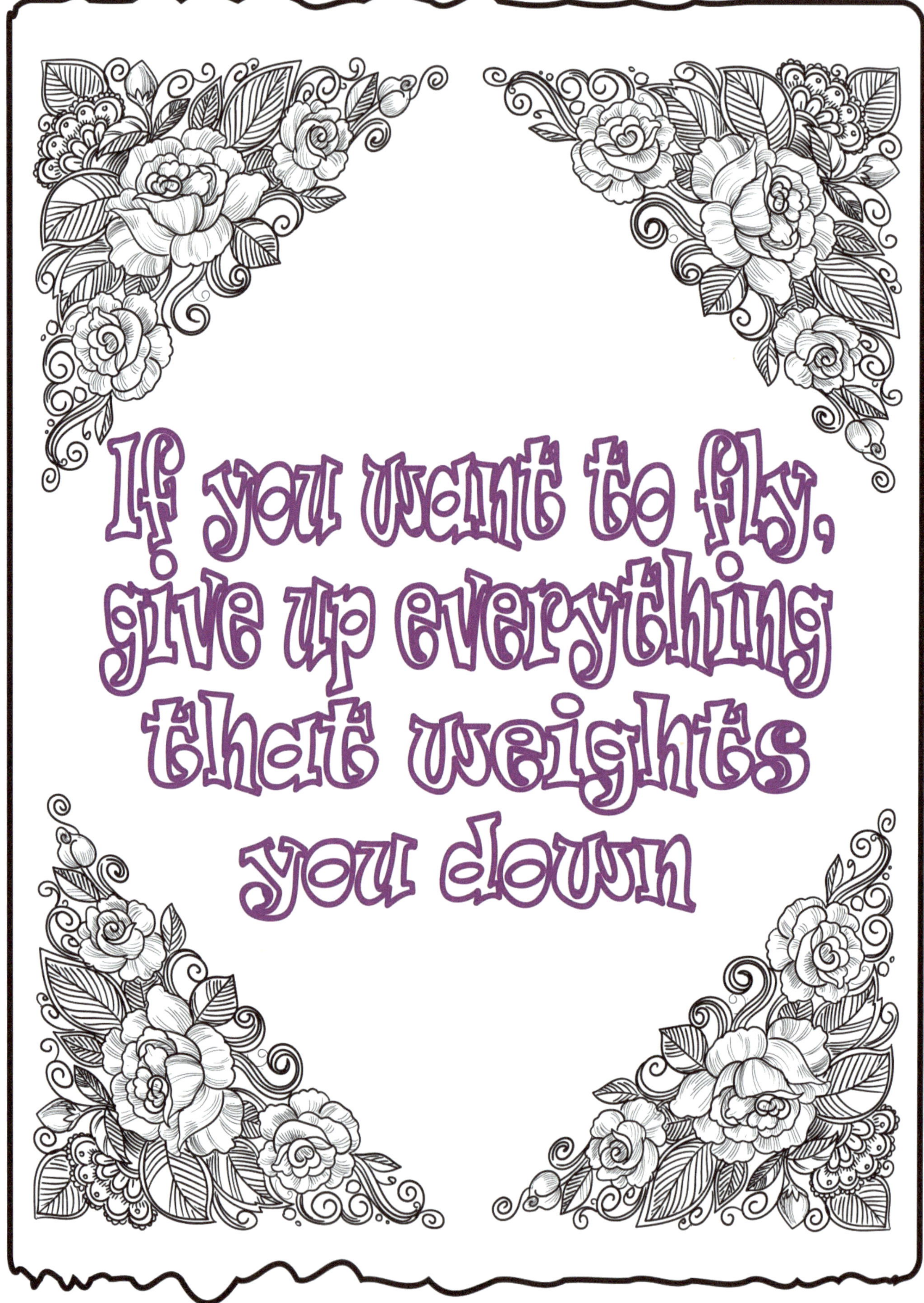

If you want to fly,
give up everything
that weights
you down

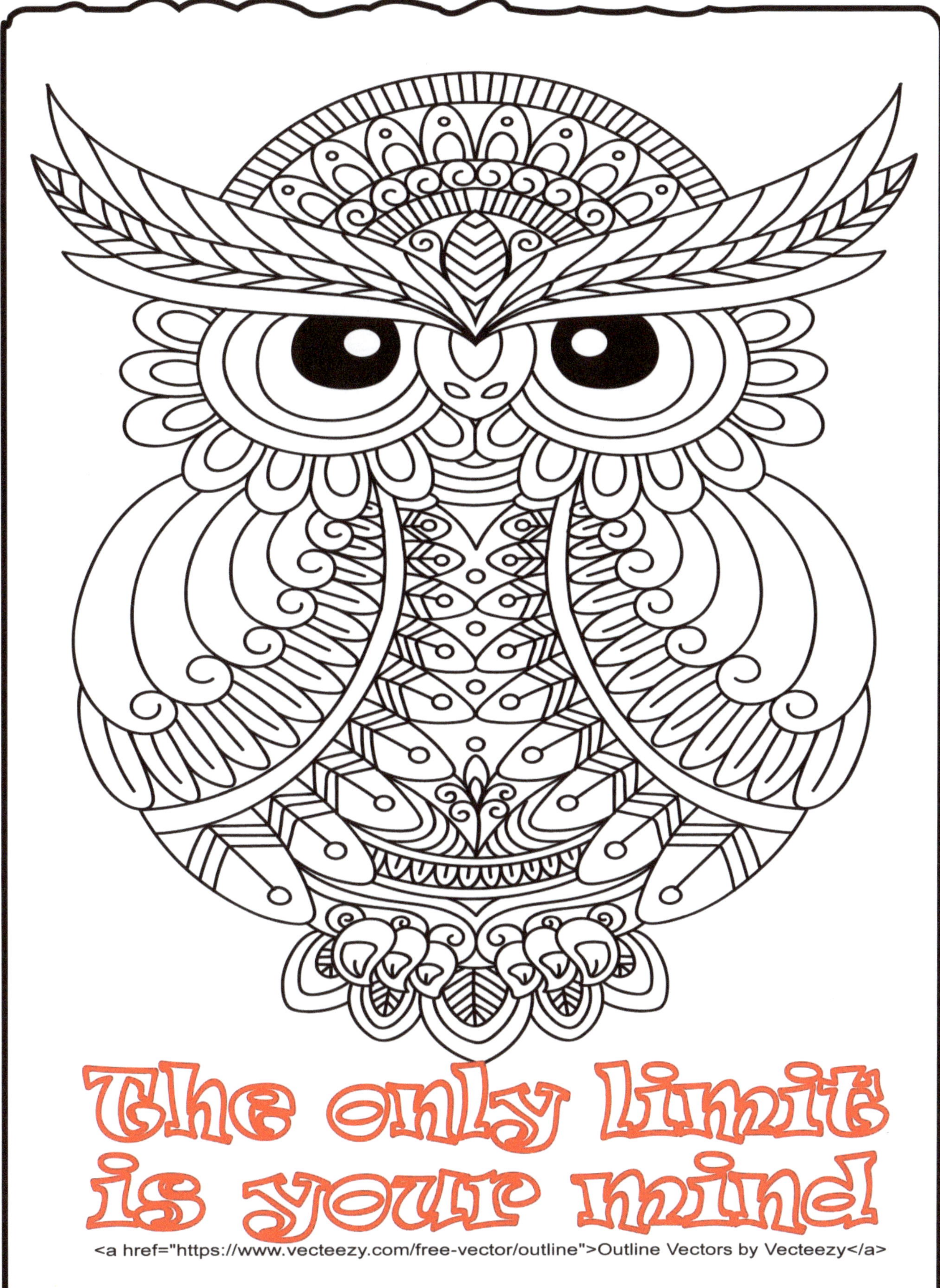

<a href="https://www.vecteezy.com/free-vector/outline">Outline Vectors by Vecteezy</a>

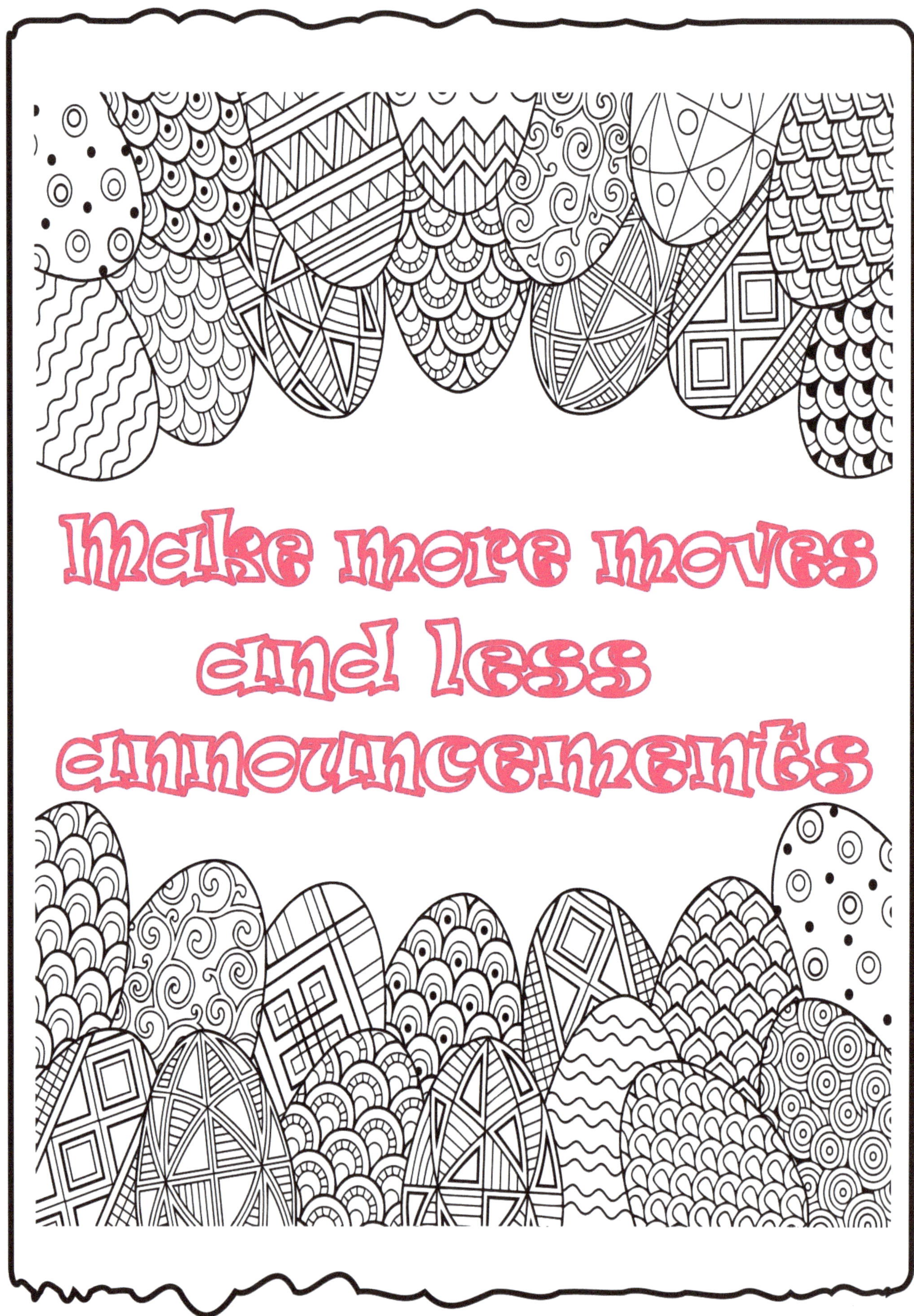
Make more moves
and less
announcements

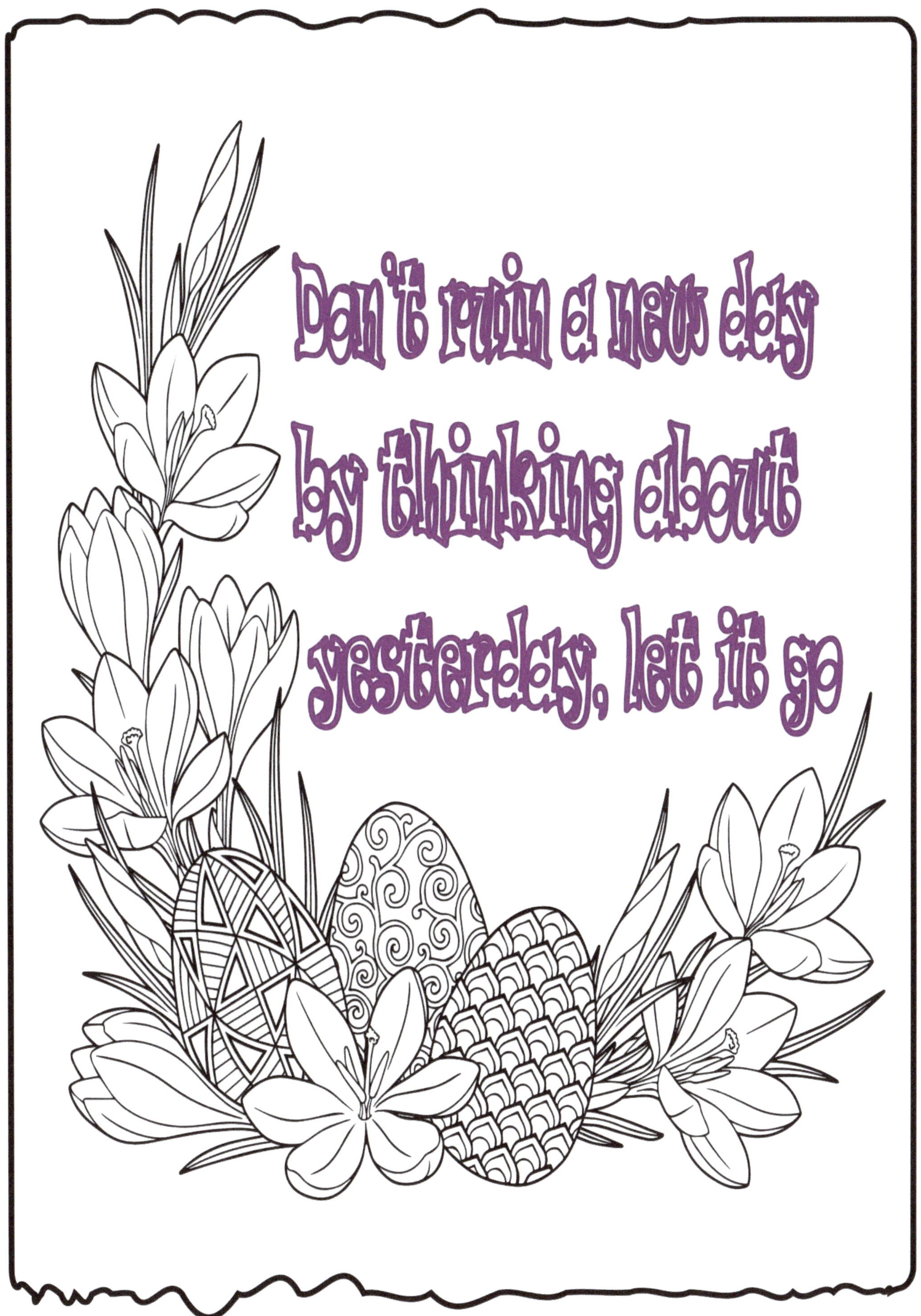
Don't ruin a new day
by thinking about
yesterday, let it go

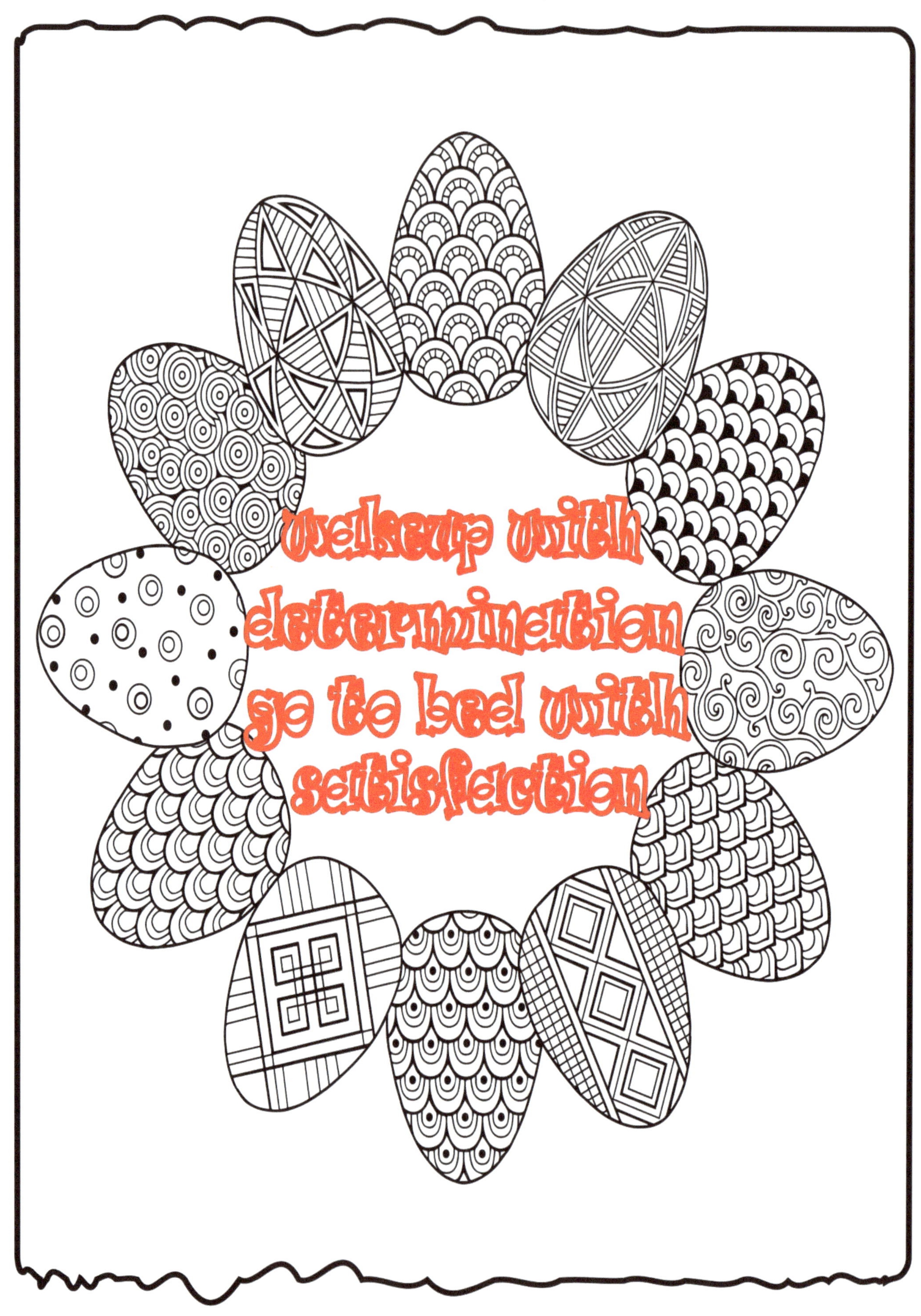

wake up with
determination
go to bed with
satisfaction

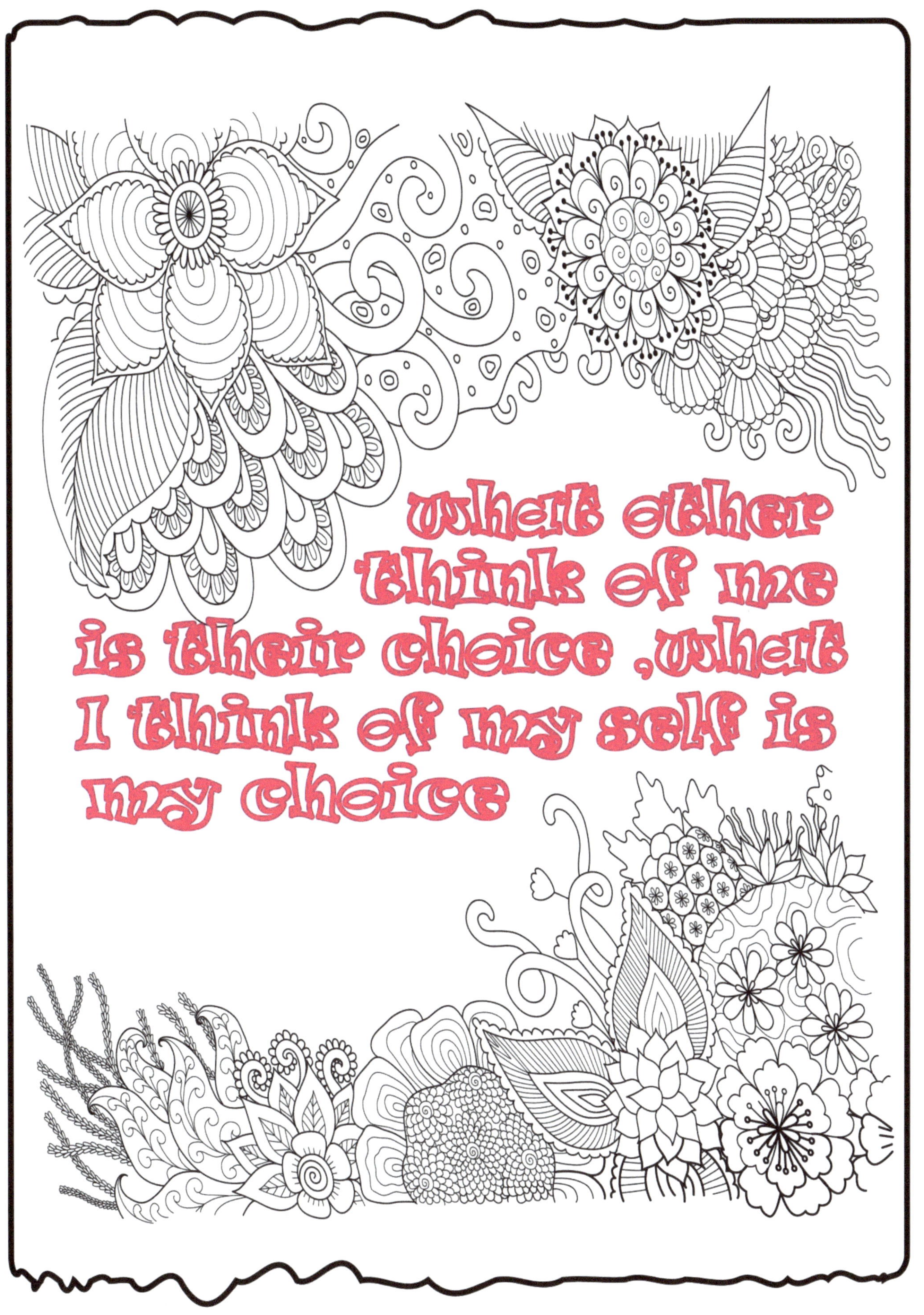

what other
think of me
is their choice , what
I think of my self is
my choice

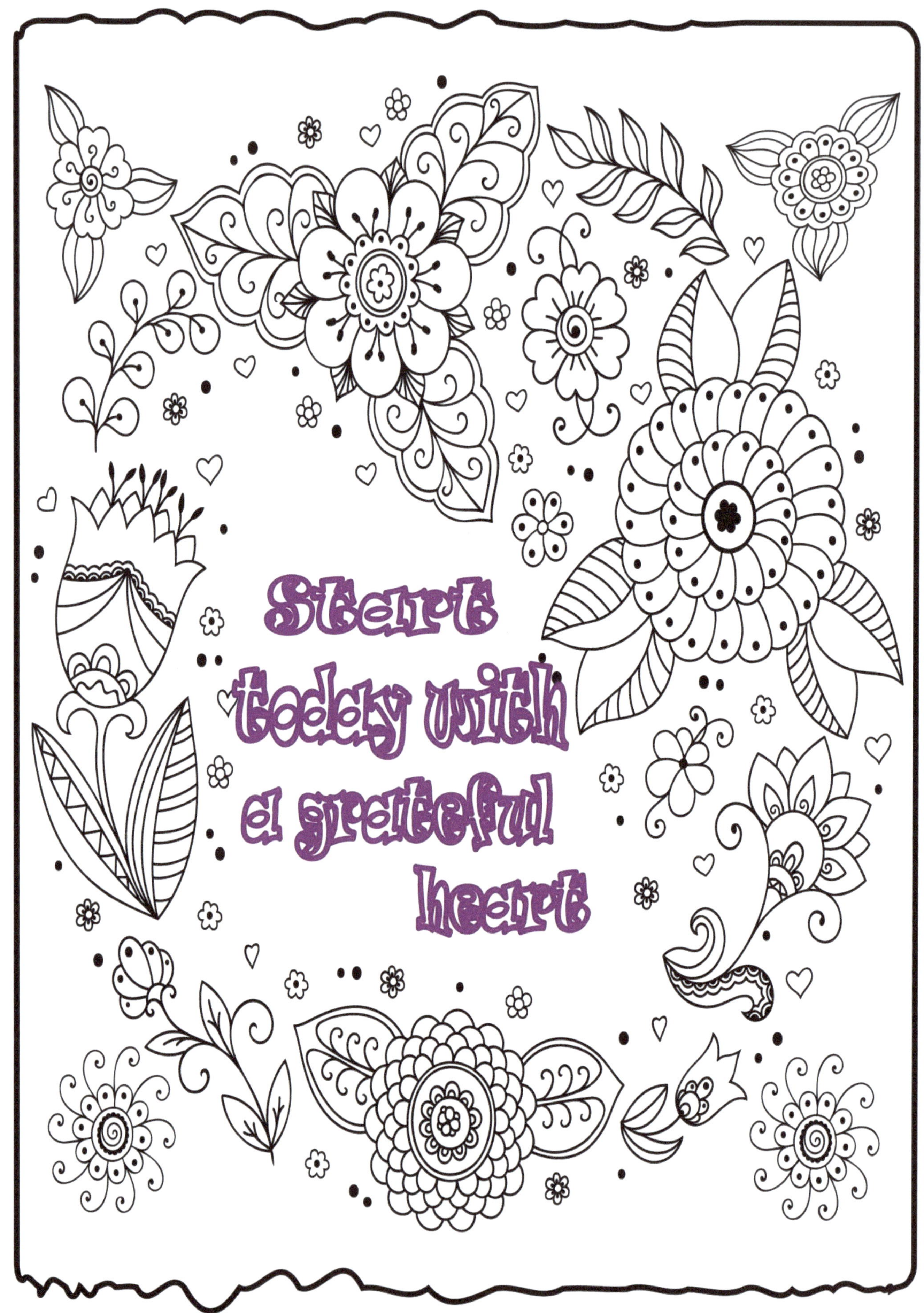
Start
today with
a grateful
heart

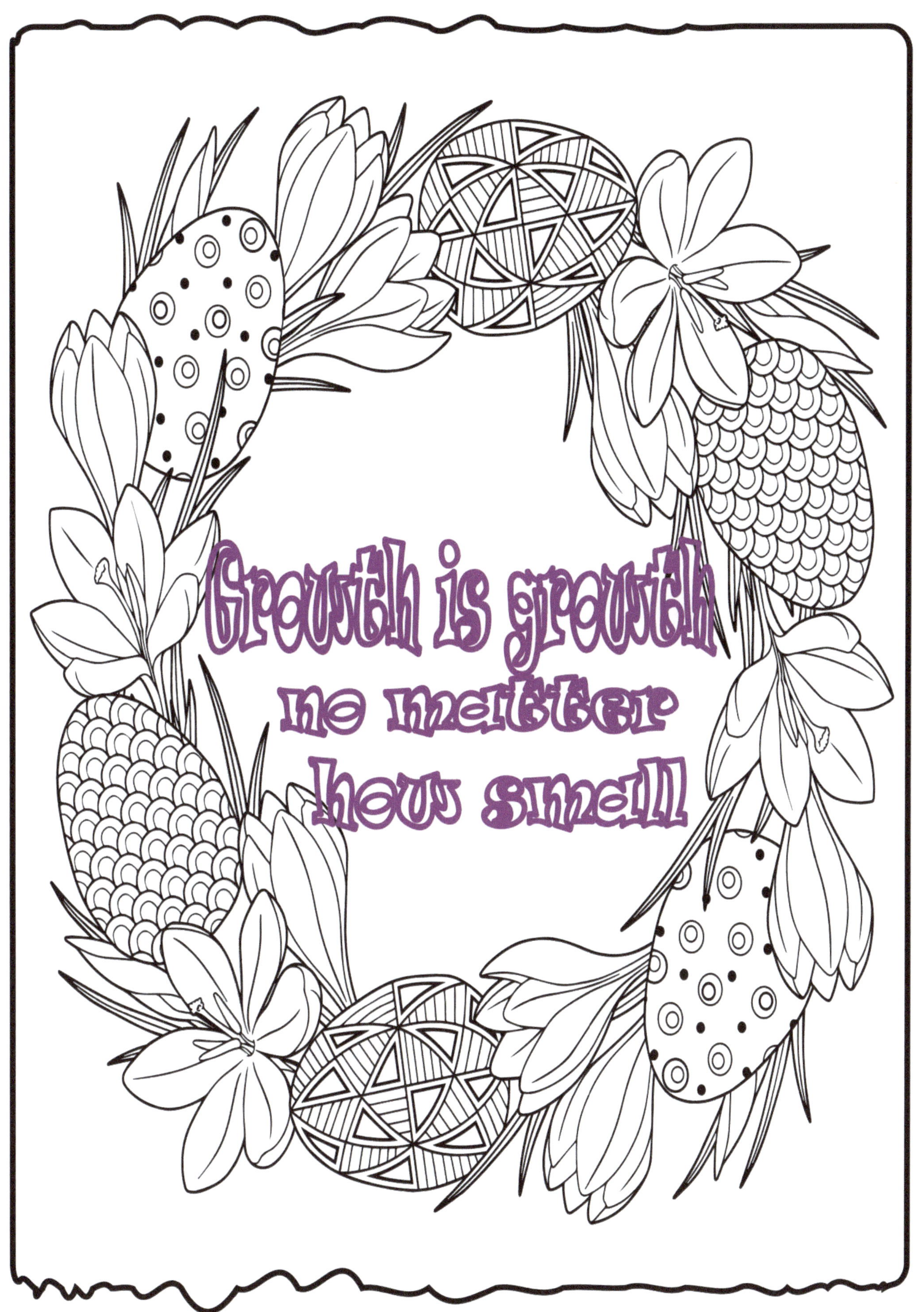

Growth is growth
no matter
how small

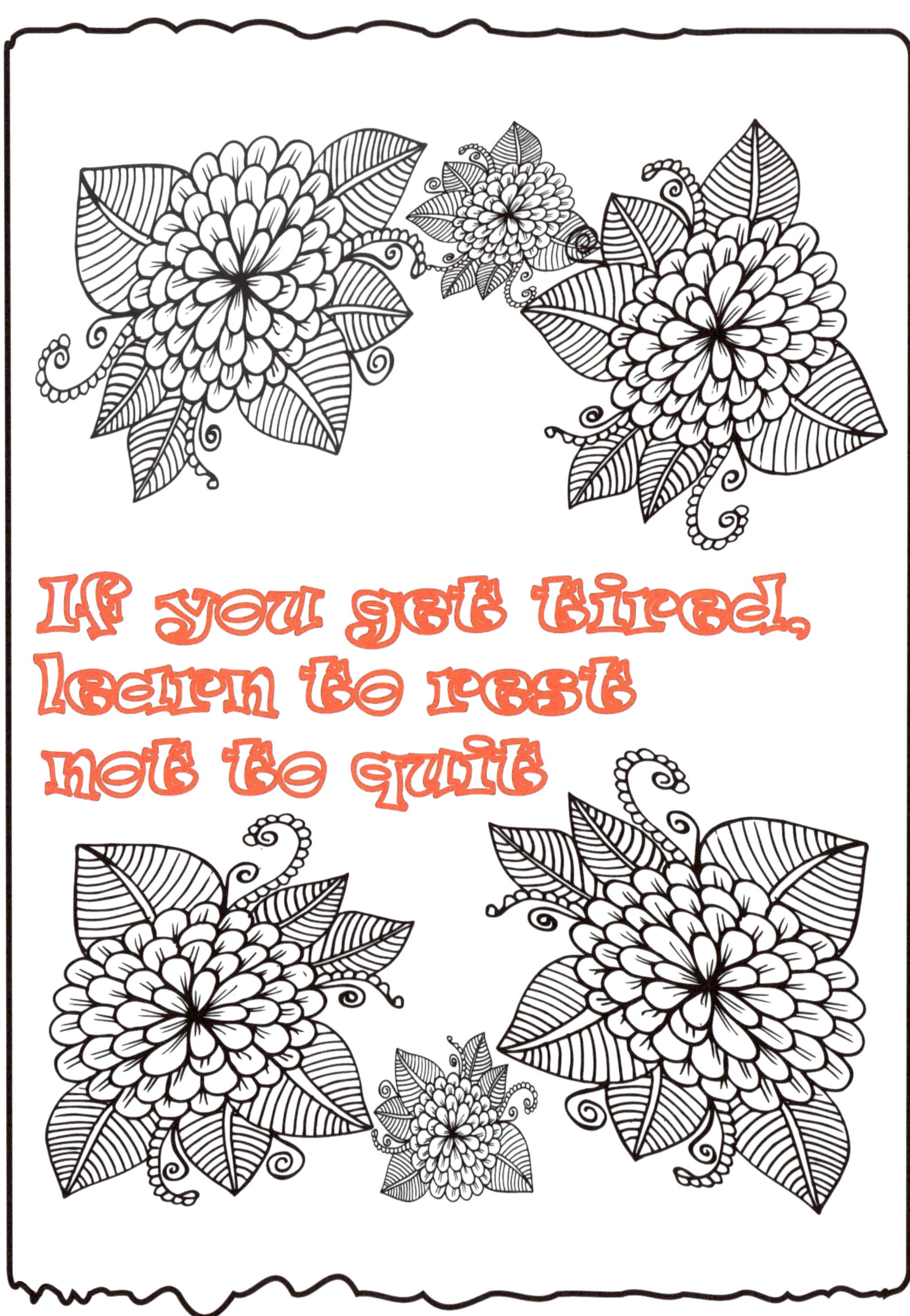

If you get tired,
learn to rest
not to quit

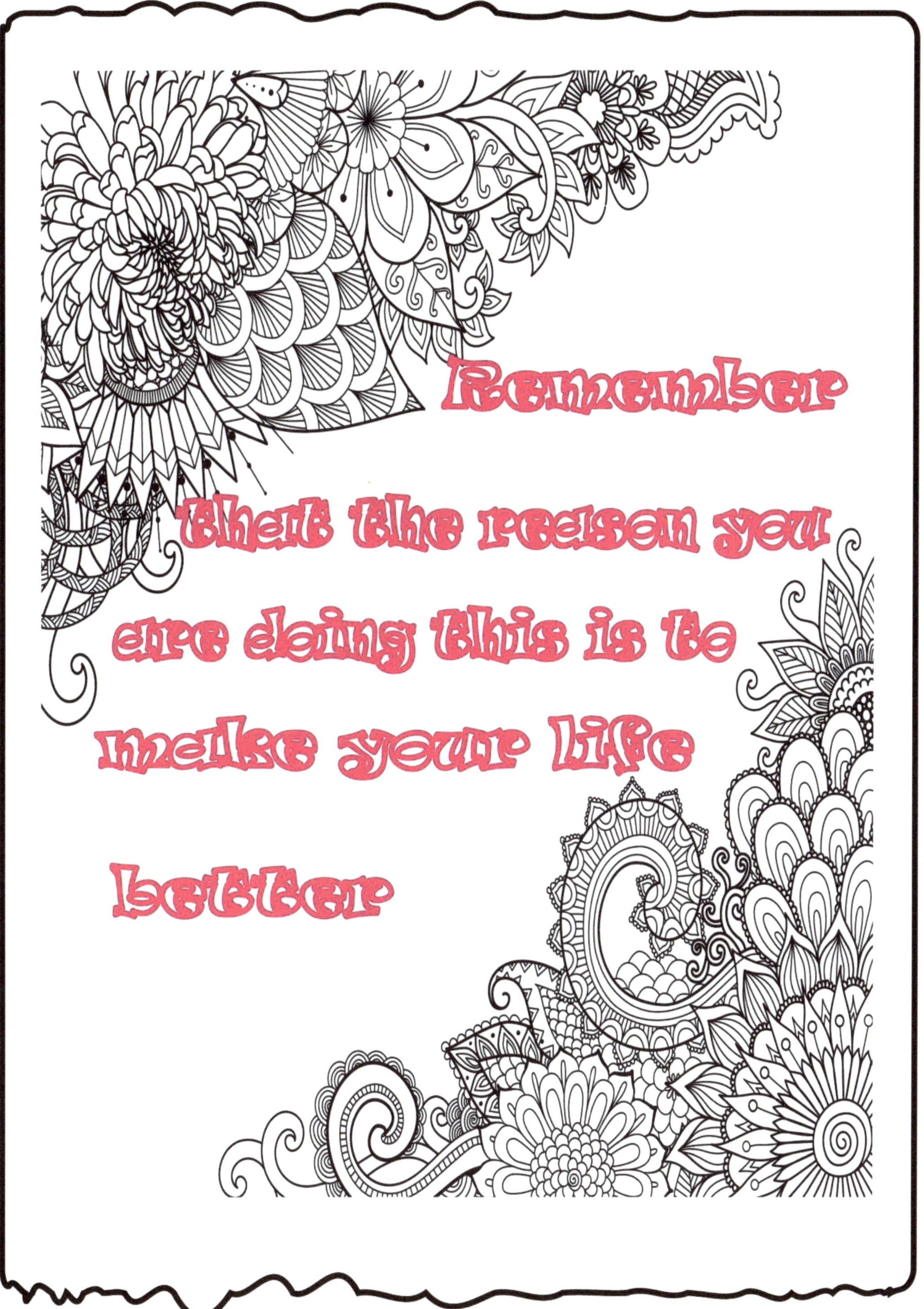

Remember
that the reason you
are doing this is to
make your life
better

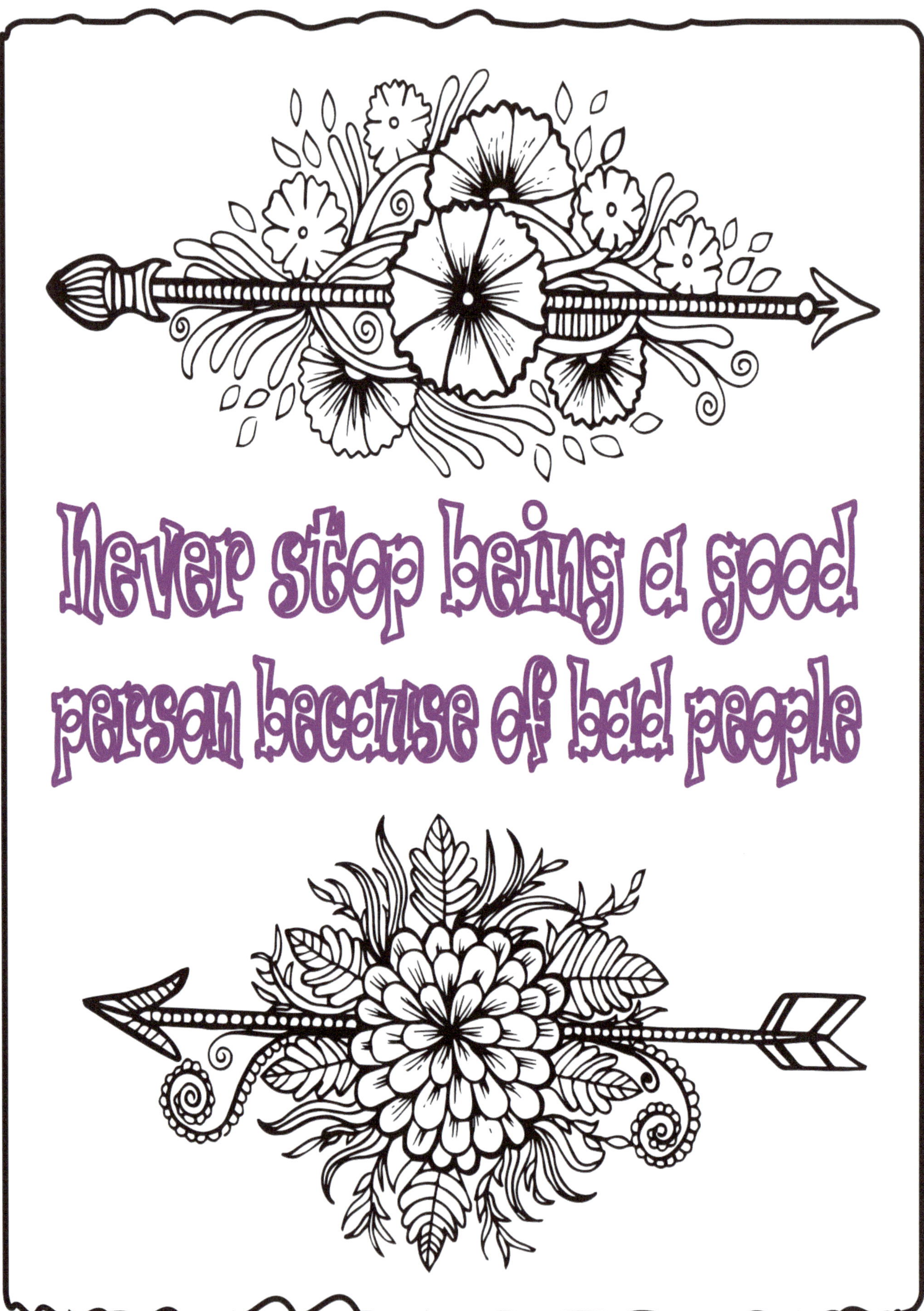

never stop being a good
person because of bad people

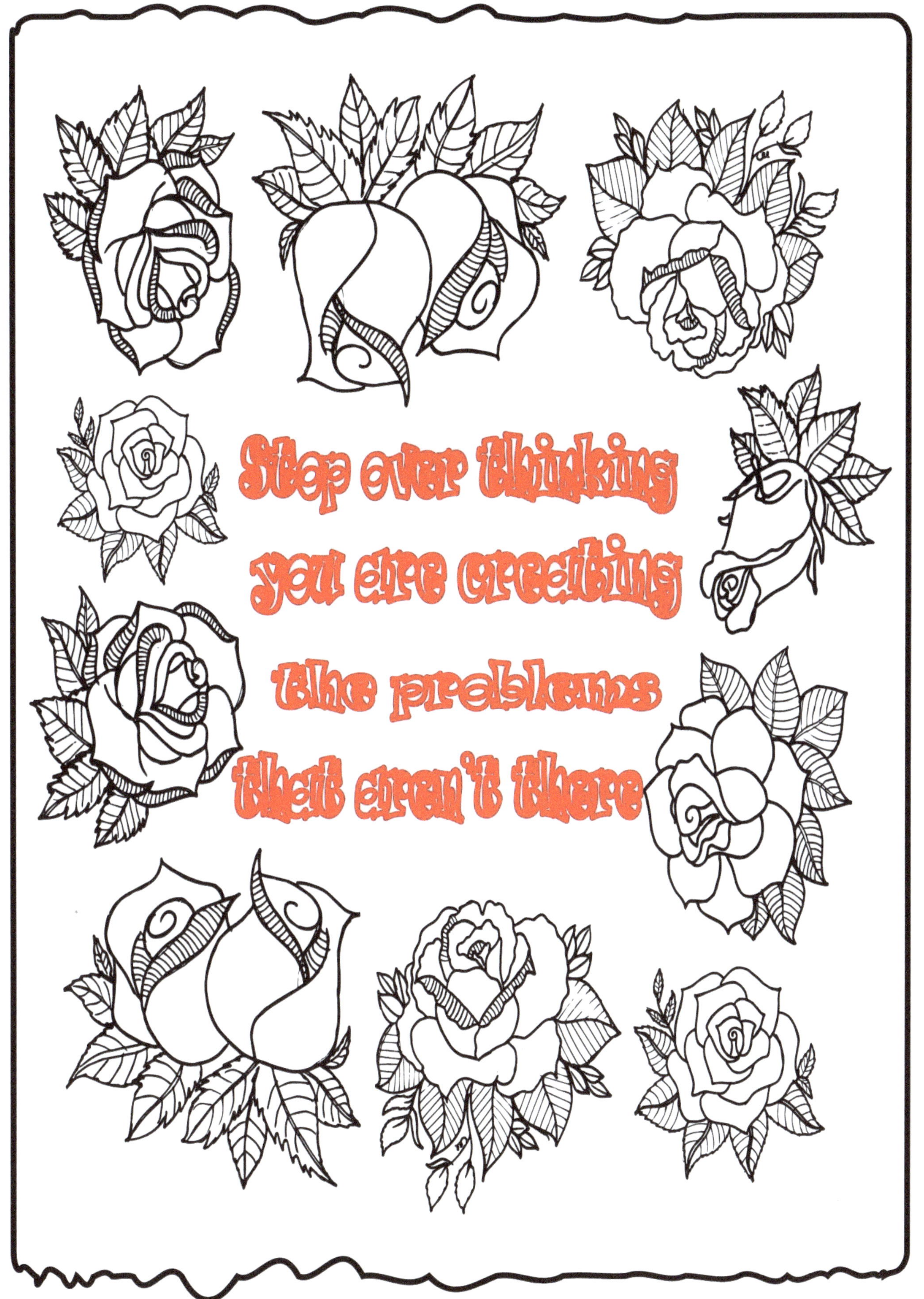
Stop over thinking
you are creating
the problems
that aren't there

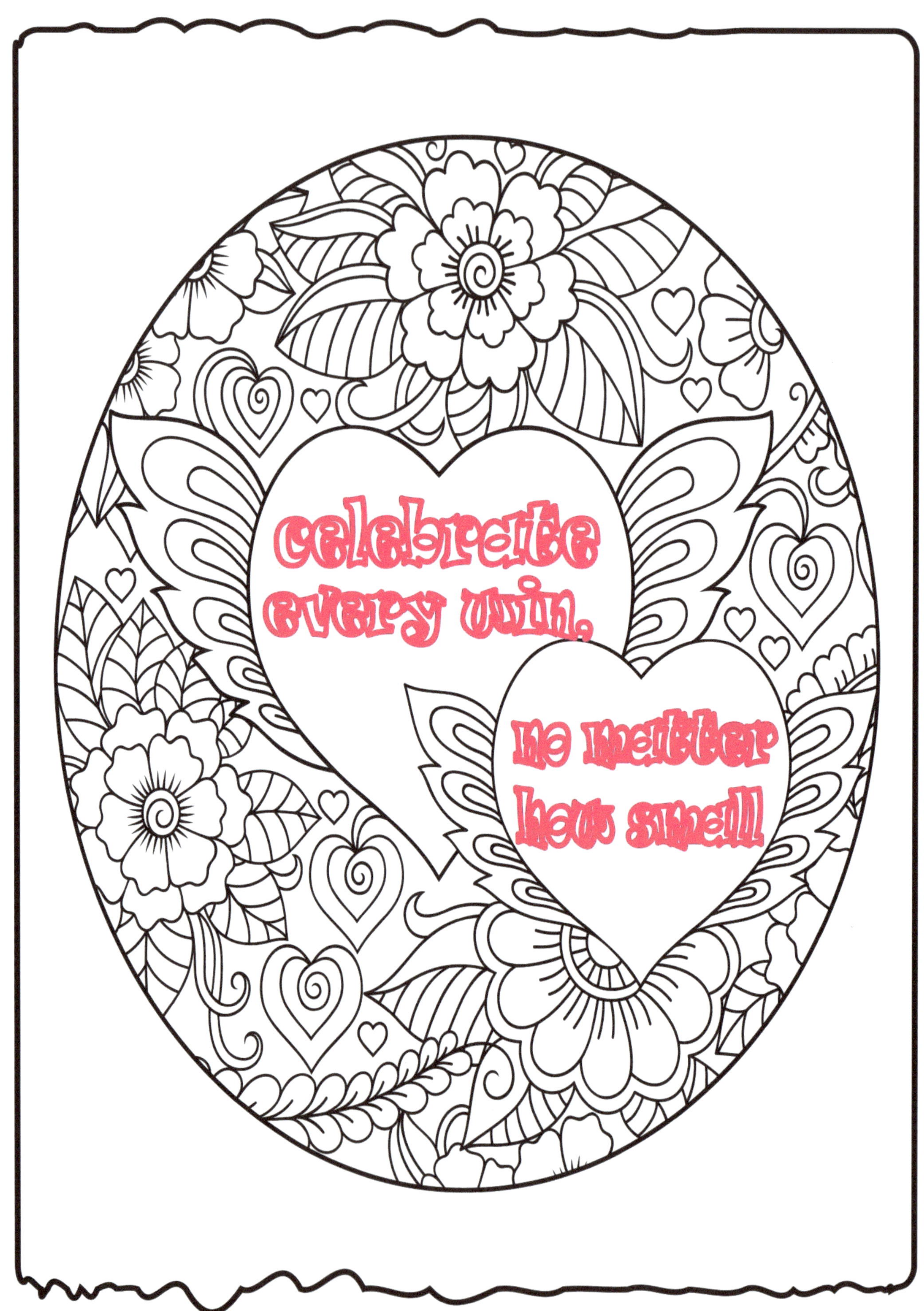

celebrate every win,
no matter how small

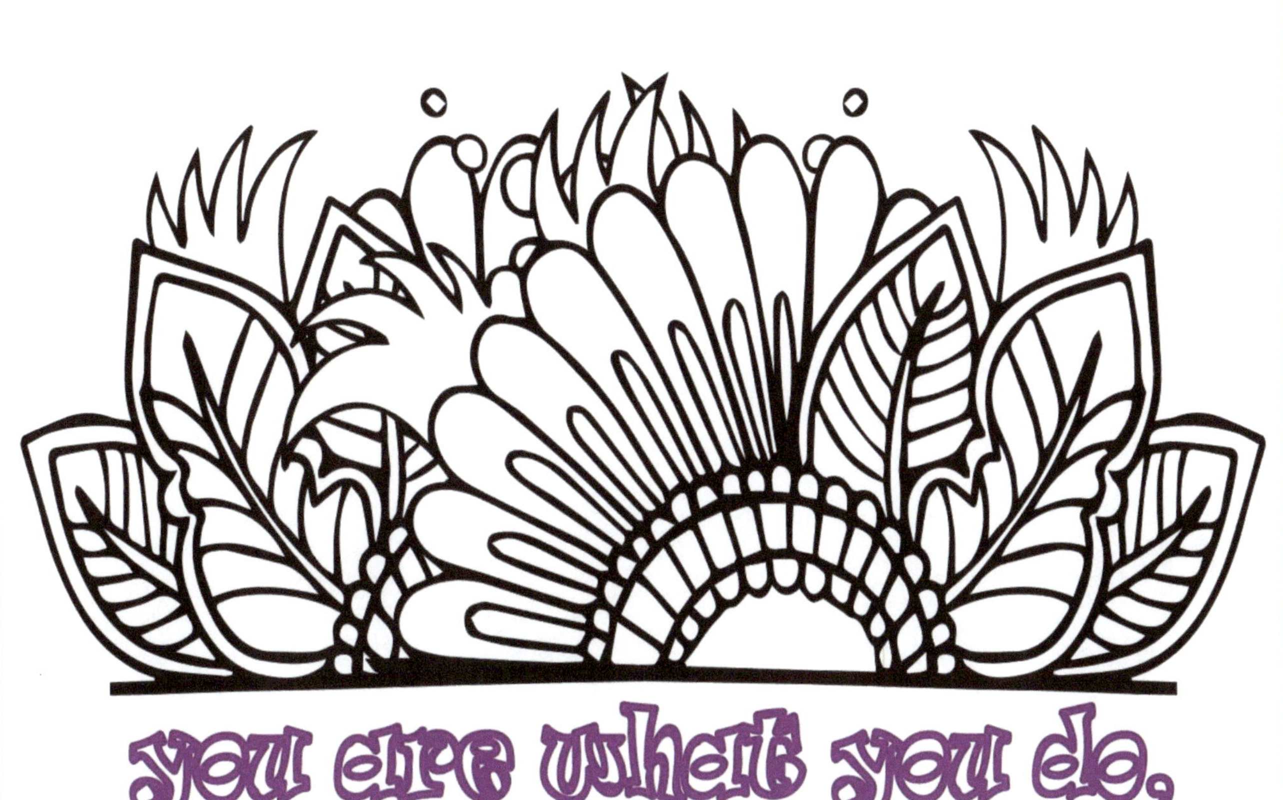

you are what you do,
not what you say
you'll do

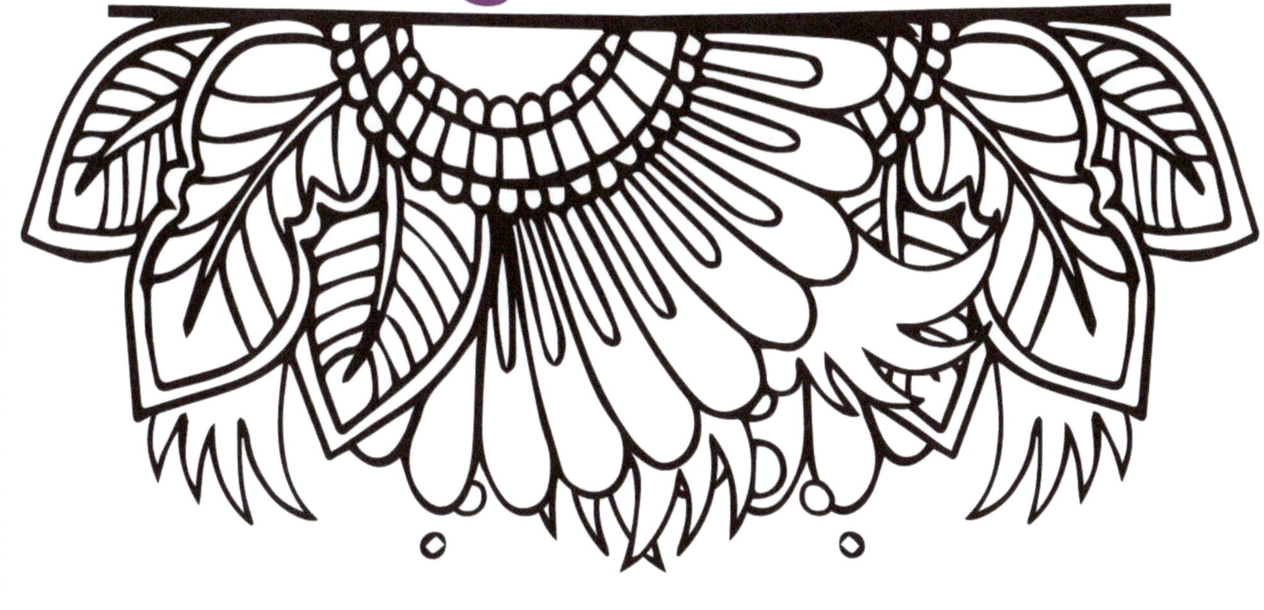

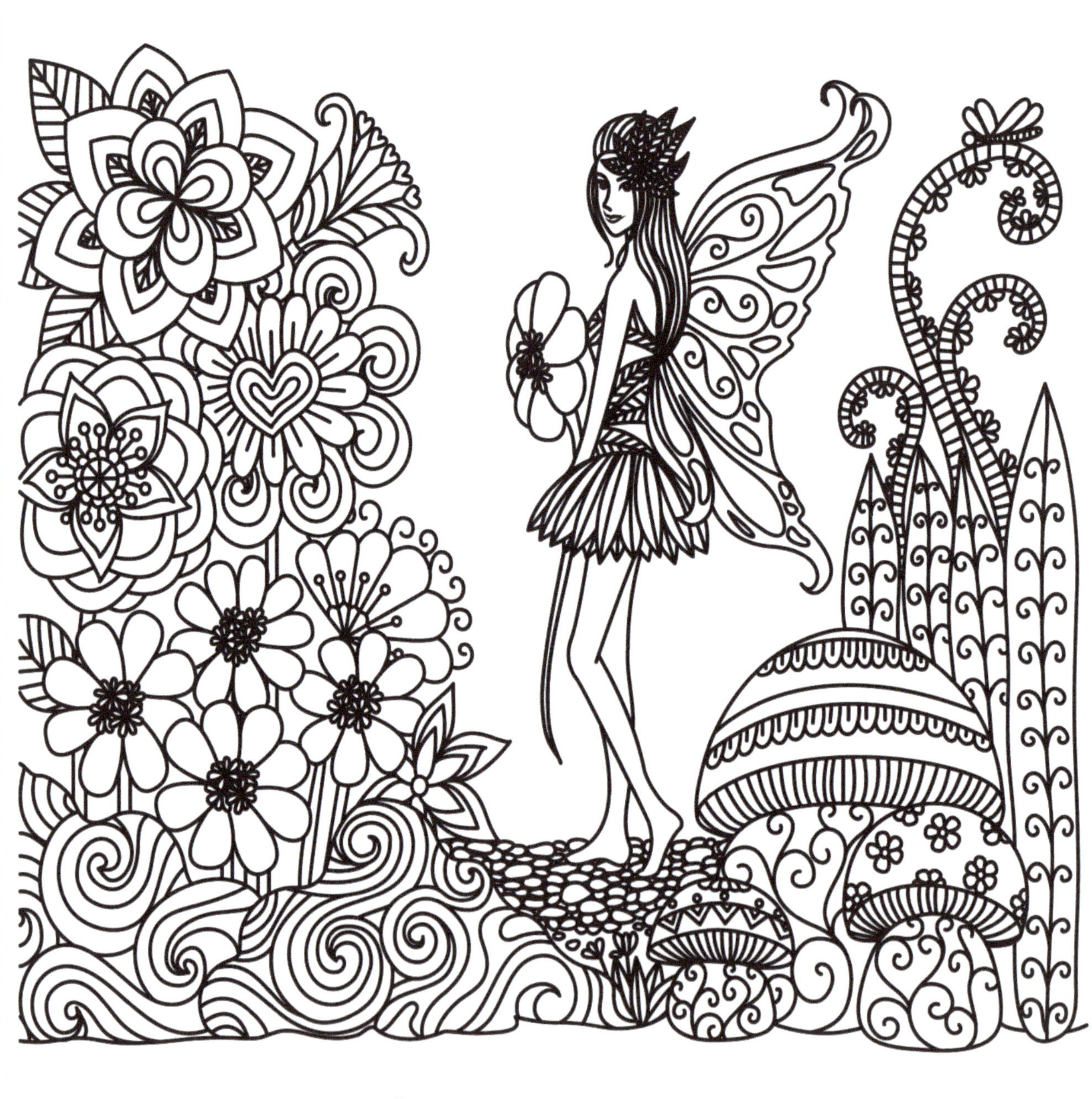

If you want to fly, give up everything that weight you down

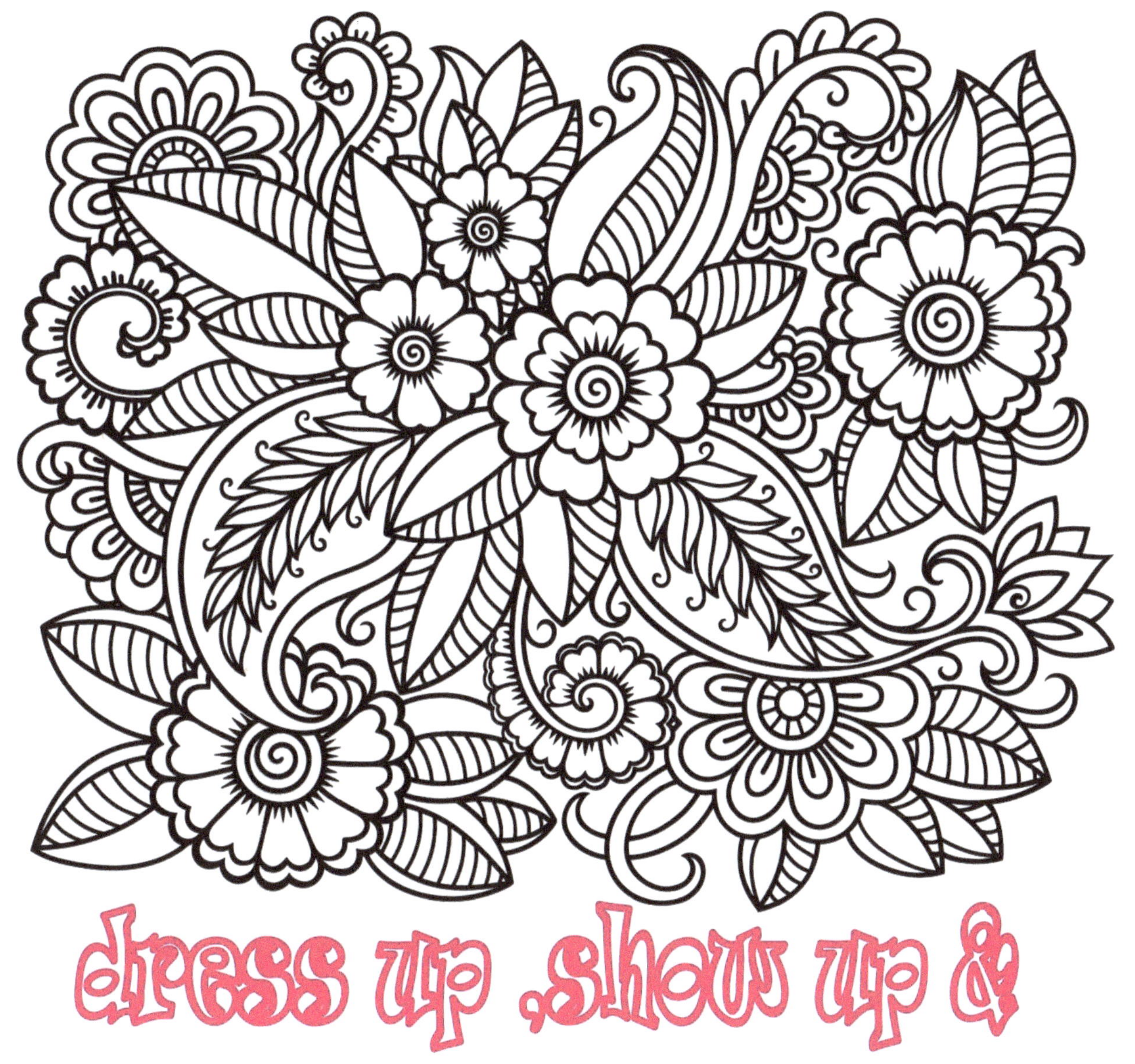
No matter how you feel
get up,
dress up ,show up &
& never give-up

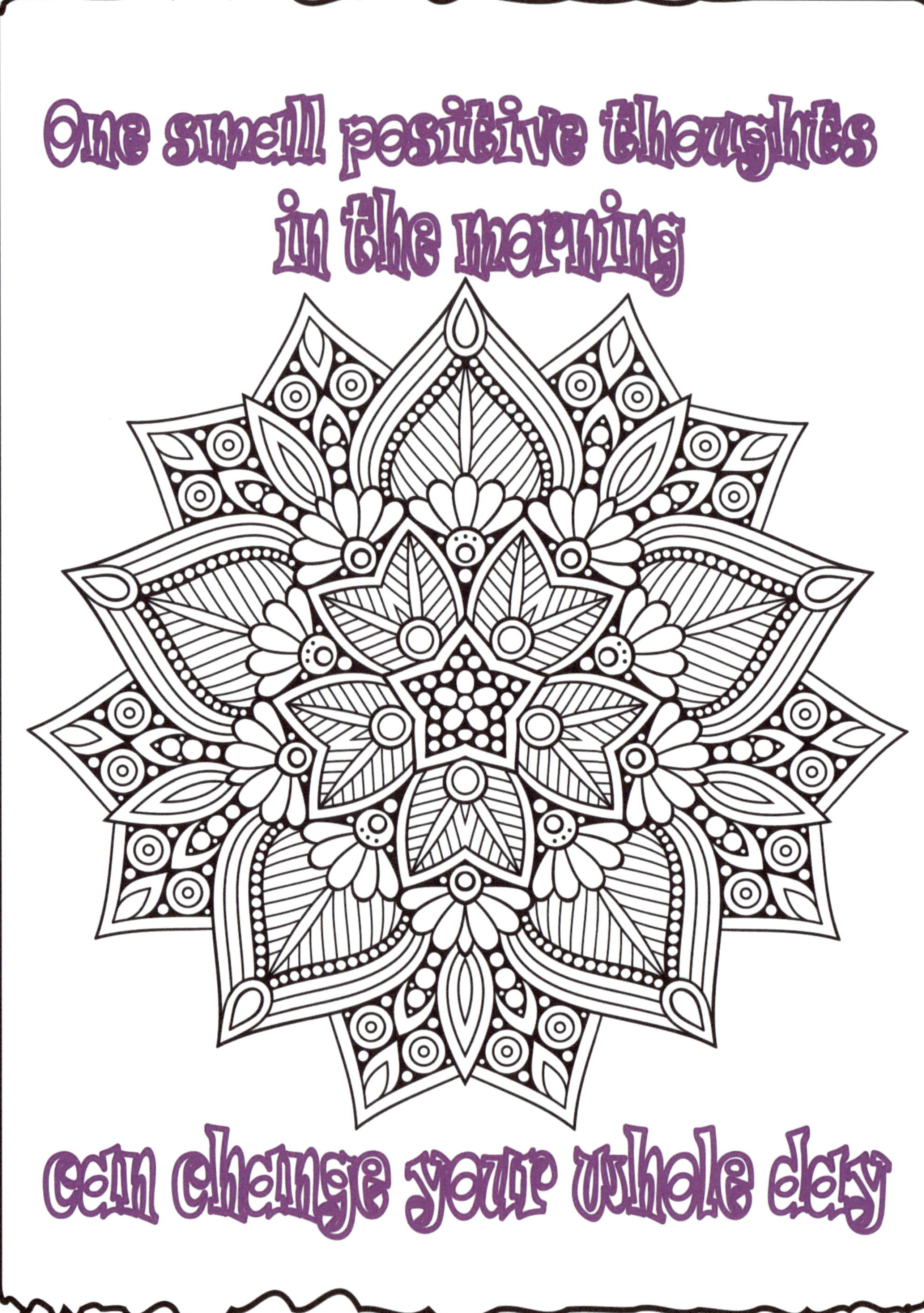
One small positive thoughts
in the morning
can change your whole day

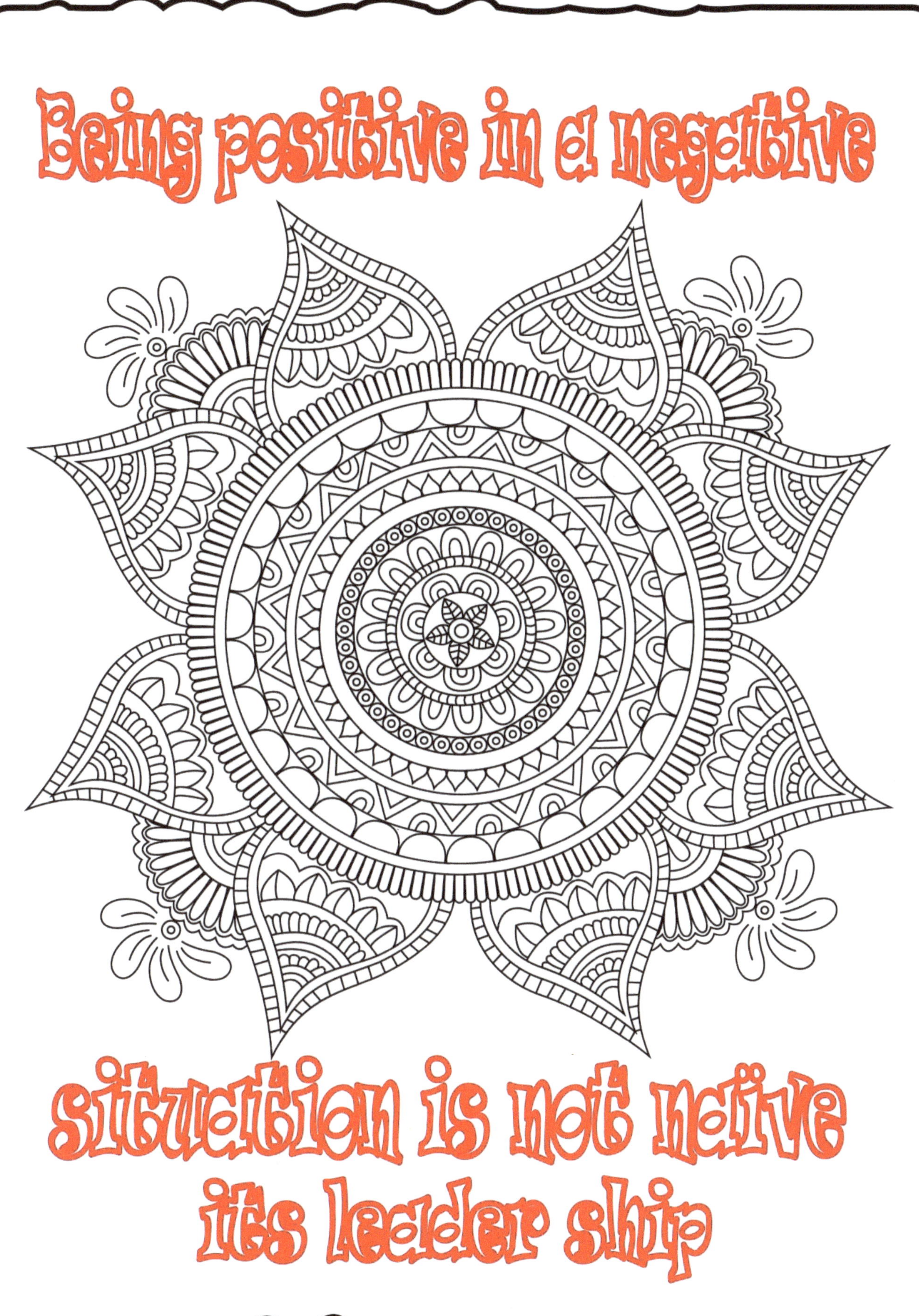

Being positive in a negative
situation is not naïve
its leader ship

Today is your opportunity

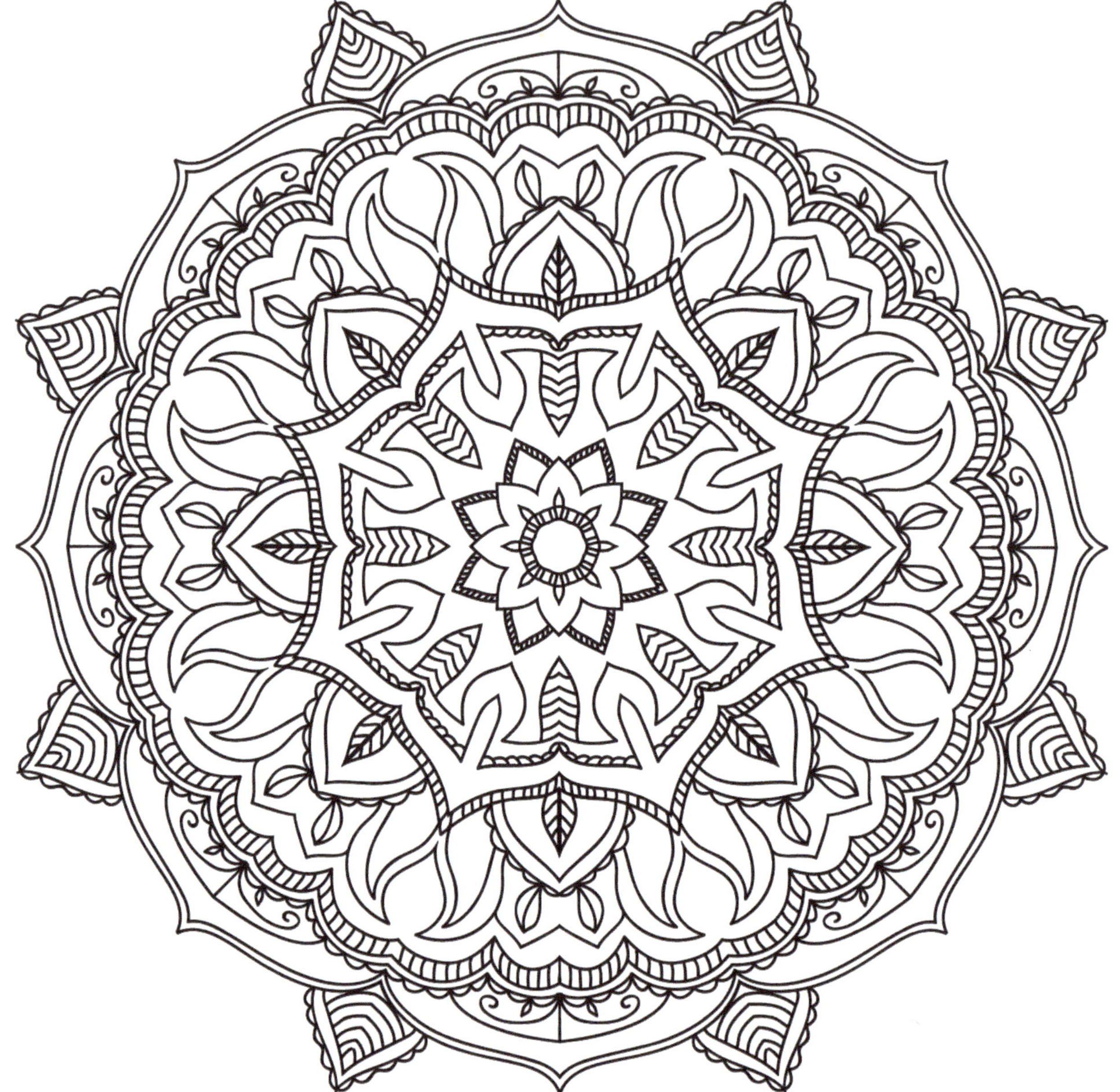

to build the tomorrow
you want

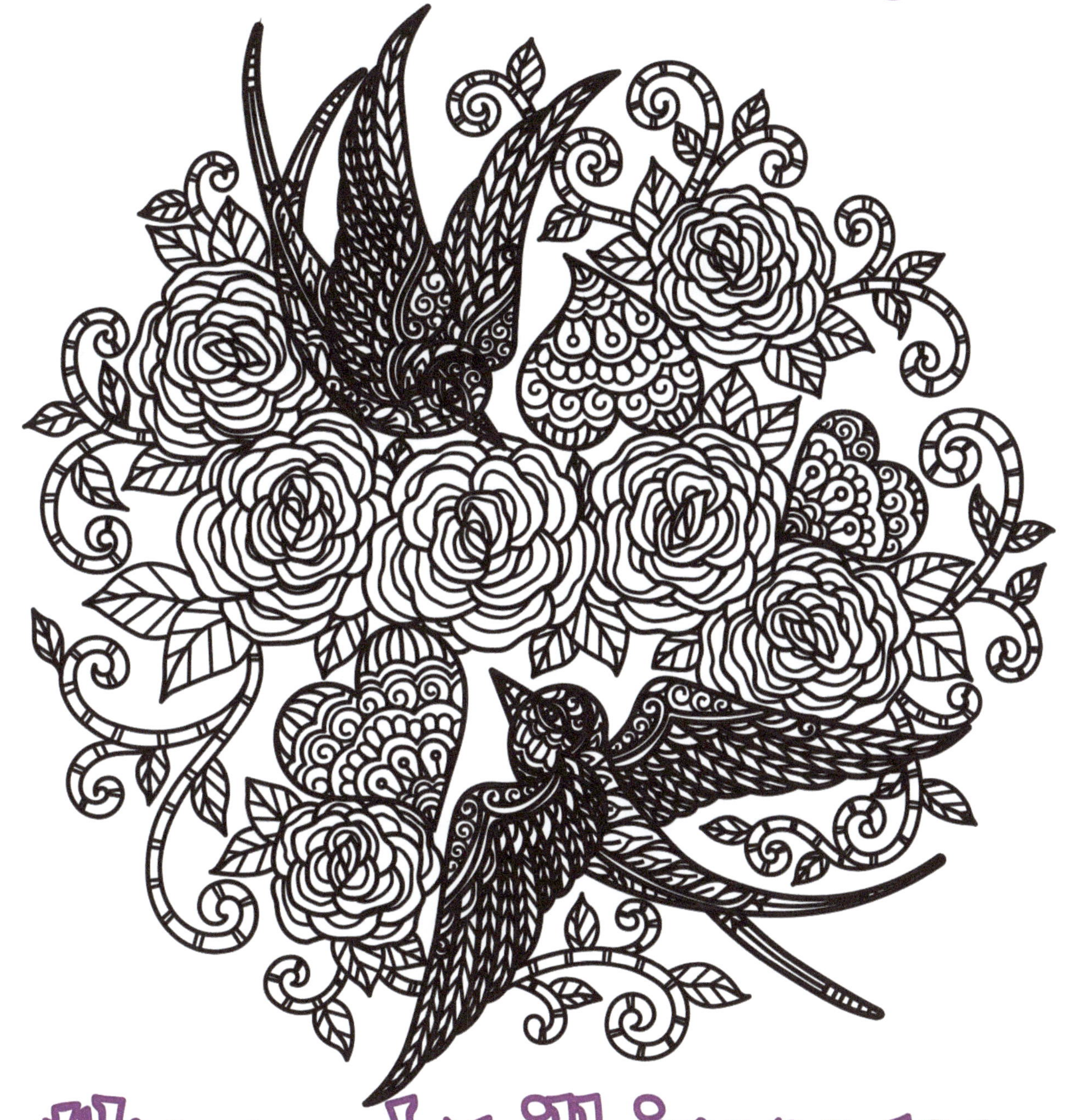

when you focus on the good,
the good will increase

www.ingramcontent.com/pod-product-compliance
Lightning Source LLC
Chambersburg PA
CBHW040049240726
48664CB00004B/1121